Obs and Gynae

PG Focus Series

Parasitic Infections in Pregnancy

Obs and Gynae
PG Focus Series
Parasitic Infections in Pregnancy

Editors

Niranjan Chavan
MD FICOG FCPS DGO DFP MICOG DICOG Diploma in Endoscopy (USA)
Professor and Unit Chief
Department of Obstetrics and Gynaecology
Lokmanya Tilak Medical College and General Hospital
Mumbai, Maharashtra, India

Komal N Chavan
MD DNB MNAMS FCPS DGO FICOG and Diploma in Reproductive Medicine (UK-SH Germany)
Senior Consultant and Unit Chief
Department of Obstetrics and Gynaecology
VN Desai Hospital
Mumbai, Maharashtra, India

Co-Editors

Sneha Venkateswaran
MBBS MS DNB FMAS
Assistant Professor
Department of Obstetrics and Gynaecology
Lokmanya Tilak Medical College and General Hospital
Mumbai, Maharashtra, India

Umme Ammara
MBBS MS DNB (Obs/Gynae)
Consultant
Department of Obstetrics and Gynaecology
Nusrah Diabetes Centre and Women's Clinic
Nagpur, Maharashtra, India

Neetika Chavan
MBBS
Intern
Krishna Institute of Medical Sciences, Karad
Mumbai, Maharashtra, India

JAYPEE

JAYPEE BROTHERS MEDICAL PUBLISHERS
The Health Sciences Publisher
New Delhi | London

Jaypee Brothers Medical Publishers (P) Ltd

Headquarters
Jaypee Brothers Medical Publishers (P) Ltd
EMCA House, 23/23-B
Ansari Road, Daryaganj
New Delhi 110 002, India
Landline: +91-11-23272143, +91-11-23272703
+91-11-23282021, +91-11-23245672
Email: jaypee@jaypeebrothers.com

Corporate Office
Jaypee Brothers Medical Publishers (P) Ltd
4838/24, Ansari Road, Daryaganj
New Delhi 110 002, India
Phone: +91-11-43574357
Fax: +91-11-43574314
Email: jaypee@jaypeebrothers.com

Overseas Office
JP Medical Ltd.
83, Victoria Street, London
SW1H 0HW (UK)
Phone: +44 20 3170 8910
Fax: +44 (0)20 3008 6180
Email: info@jpmedpub.com

Website: www.jaypeebrothers.com
Website: www.jaypeedigital.com

Inquiries for bulk sales may be solicited at: jaypee@jaypeebrothers.com

Obs and Gynae PG Focus Series: Parasitic Infections in Pregnancy

First Edition: **2025**

ISBN: 978-93-6616-476-2

Printed in India

Preface

Pregnancy represents a unique physiological state where the health of both the mother and the developing fetus must be carefully balanced. While advancements in maternal and fetal care have significantly improved outcomes in many regions, pregnant women remain vulnerable to a range of infections, including parasitic diseases. These infections not only pose significant health risks to the mother but can also result in serious complications, affecting fetal development and long-term child health.

This textbook, *Parasitic Infections in Pregnancy,* aims to provide an in-depth and comprehensive understanding of the various parasitic infections that can affect pregnant women. It seeks to bridge the gap between the medical, clinical, and parasitological sciences, providing both foundational knowledge and practical guidelines for managing these infections in a clinical setting.

As a textbook designed for postgraduate students, clinicians, and researchers, this volume aims to stimulate a multidisciplinary approach to understanding and managing parasitic infections in pregnancy. It will serve as a vital resource for those involved in maternal health, infectious disease control, and global health efforts. The content reflects the most recent advances in the field, incorporating new research findings and clinical insights to ensure that readers are equipped with up-to-date information in an ever-evolving field of medicine.

We hope this textbook contributes to a better understanding of the crucial intersection between parasitic infections and pregnancy and fosters improved outcomes for both maternal and child health worldwide.

Editors
Niranjan Chavan
Komal N Chavan

Co-Editors
Sneha Venkateswaran
Umme Ammara
Neetika Chavan

Acknowledgments

We express our gratitude to all those who contributed to the completion of this book on *Parasitic Infections in Pregnancy*. This endeavor would not have been possible without the constant support of many individuals.

We are thankful to all the authors and co-authors for sharing their expertise and commitment to producing a resource of the highest standards.

We are grateful to our mentors and colleagues, whose valuable guidance helped us form the structure and contents of this book.

Our deepest gratitude to our families and friends for their unwavering support, patience, and encouragement during the demanding phases of this project have been our greatest strength.

We acknowledge the support of Shri Jitendar P Vij (Group Chairman) and Mr Ankit Vij (Managing Director) of M/s Jaypee Brothers Medical Publishers (P) Ltd, New Delhi, India, in publishing the book and their associates, particularly Ms Chetna Malhotra (Senior Director—Professional Publishing, Marketing, and Business Development), Ms Kritika Dua (Senior Commissioning Editor), and Ms Pragati Singh (Development Editor), who have been prompt, efficient, and most helpful.

Lastly, we hope that the postgraduate students find this book useful in their examinations and teachers for a quick revision. We also hope this book serves as a valuable resource, contributing to the betterment of patient care and surgical practice to the practicing obstetricians and gynaecologists.

Thank you all for being a part of this journey.

Contents

CHAPTER 1

Introduction

Parasitic infections are fairly common and affect millions of pregnant women throughout the world. Clinicians increasingly are confronted with parasitic infections such as malaria, trypanosomiasis, and schistosomiasis, because of the increase in international travel. These infections lead directly and indirectly to a spectrum of adverse maternal and fetal/placental effects. However, most clinicians are inexperienced in the diagnosis and treatment of these cases. Obstetricians should have knowledge of the biology, life cycle, and clinical manifestations of each parasite. The decision to treat a parasitic infection during pregnancy is a difficult risk-benefit calculation based on knowledge of the associated morbidity and mortality, and the toxic effects of the antiparasitic drug. Because no definitive data are available on the safety of most antiparasitic drugs in pregnancy, drug therapy is indicated only in life-threatening situations or when the benefits of the drug clearly exceed the risks. The pregnant woman should be informed of the risks of treating a parasitic disease during pregnancy. Withholding treatment is appropriate when the infection does not pose an immediate threat to the mother or fetus.

This monogram summarizes the clinical aspects, treatment, and potential toxicity of treatment for common parasitic infections that might be encountered during pregnancy.

CHAPTER 2

Pathophysiology of Parasitic Infections

INTRODUCTION

- *Parasitic infection:* It is the asymptomatic invasion of the parasite in a host's body.
- *Parasitic disease:* It refers to the clinical manifestations along with infection of the parasite.

A general overview of the sources of infection of various parasitic infections and their clinical manifestations is given in this chapter. Subsequent chapters will deal in greater detail regarding the individual parasites, their life cycle, modes of transmission, and management methods in pregnant and lactating women.

SOURCES OF INFECTION

The major sources of infection are as follows:

- *Soil:*
  - Embryonated eggs present in the soil may be ingested, for example, roundworm.
  - Larvae present in the soil may penetrate through the skin, for example, *Strongyloides stercoralis* and hookworm.
- *Water:*
  - Swallowing of infective forms (like cysts of amoeba) from contaminated water.
  - Swallowing of the intermediate host (like guinea worm in Cyclops infection).
  - Penetration of infective larvae in the water through exposed skin, for example, a cercarial form of schistosomes.
- *Food:*
  - Fecal contamination of food with cysts of amoebae, pinworm, and oocysts of toxoplasma.
  - Some types of meat may contain infective larvae.
- *Insect vectors:*
  - Biological vectors—mosquitoes, sandflies, reduviid bugs, and ticks.
  - Mechanical vectors—housefly.
- *Animals:*
  - Cows—beef tapeworm (*Taenia saginata*)
  - Pig—pork tapeworm (*Taenia solium*)

    - Dog—hydatid disease (Echinococcosis)
    - Cat—toxoplasmosis
    - Fish—fish tapeworm (*Diphyllobothrium latum*)
- *Vertical transmission*: Congenital toxoplasmosis and congenital malaria
- *Autoinfection*:
    - Finger-to-mouth transmission, e.g., pinworm.
    - Intestinal reinfection, e.g., *Strongyloides stercoralis*.

CLINICAL MANIFESTATIONS

The clinical manifestations of a parasitic disease depend upon various factors. These include:

- Degree of parasitemia
- Ability of the parasite to escape host immune responses[1]
- Host immunity level
- Host nutritional status
- Systemic or local responses depend on the type of parasite: protozoa usually cause systemic response, while local responses are more commonly seen with worms.

Common signs and symptoms of parasitic disease:

- *Fever:* This is the most common symptom of any parasitic disease. The degree and type of fever largely depend on the species, stage of life cycle, and load of parasitemia. For example, in the disease caused by the protozoan parasite *Plasmodium falciparum*, the fever paroxysms are periodical when the mature erythrocytic schizonts rupture and release schizonts and fragments of erythrocytes into the bloodstream. This is usually accompanied by rigor.
- *Anemia:* This is caused in varying degrees and types by various parasites **(Table 1)**.
- *Diarrhea:* There are various mechanisms for the development of diarrhea in parasitic infections. These include:
    - Mechanical damages due to local intestinal lesions[2]
    - Allergic reactions

TABLE 1: Types of parasites with pathophysiology of anemia.[2]

Adult hookworm	Chronic anemia	The hookworms parasitize the intestine and suck blood; therefore, the host suffers from chronic blood loss anemia (microcytic hypochromic)
Plasmodium species	Hemolytic anemia	These destroy the host erythrocytes, cause hypersplenism, and suppress hematopoiesis. Thus, the host suffers from hemolytic anemia
Leishmania donovani	Immune hemolysis	These colonize in the splenic macrophage system and cause hyperplasia of the mononuclear phagocytic system

TABLE 2: Liver damage in parasitic diseases.[3]

Parasite	*Liver damage*
Schistosoma japonicum	Acute inflammatory state, significant tenderness when the egg granulomas are formed
Clonorchis sinensis	Lives in a hepatobiliary duct, which causes hepatomegaly predominantly on the left side. May also cause cholestasis and present with jaundice
Entamoeba histolytica	Hepatic amoebiasis
Echinococcus granulosus	Space occupying liver cysts

- Toxic effects of metabolites and secretions of parasites
- Intestinal dysfunction

- *Allergic response:* The immune response triggered by parasitic infections stimulates the host to produce immunoglobulin E (IgE). IgE adheres to mast cells and basophils. Upon repeat infection, the mast cells and basophils undergo degranulation. Various molecules like histamine and other chemokines are released which then lead to classic manifestations of anaphylaxis.
- *Impaired nutrition status:* The parasites are known to live off the hosts' nutrients, and this may cause nutritional deficiencies and their corresponding manifestations in the host. Specific nutritional deficiencies and manifestations are discussed in further chapters.
- *Liver damage*: The liver is one of the most commonly affected organs in parasitic diseases, mechanisms of these are enumerated in **Table 2**.
- *Central nervous system (CNS) affection:* These may be:
  - Cerebral space-occupying lesions such as amoebic brain abscesses, neurocysticercosis, and schistosomiasis.
  - Encephalitis
  - Meningitis

REFERENCES

1. Rijken MJ, McGready R, Boel ME, et al. Malaria in Pregnancy in the Asia-Pacific region. Lancet Infect Dis. 2012;12:75-88.
2. Murray P, Baron E, Pfaller M, et al. Manual of Clinical Microbiology. 2007;9.
3. Friedman JF, Mital P, Kanzaria HK, et al. Schistosomiasis and Pregnancy. Trends Parasitol. 2007;23:159-64.

CHAPTER 3

Immunology of Parasites and Pregnancy

INTRODUCTION

The immune response to parasitic infection leads to a complex interplay with the immune changes of pregnancy. CD4-T cells can differentiate into one of two types of T-helper cells, a T-helper cell type 1 (Th1) or a T-helper cell type 2 (Th2) cell. Th1 cells activate a cytotoxic response through cytokines, including interferon-gamma (IFN-γ), tumor necrosis factor-alpha (TNF-α), and interleukin (IL)-12.[1] The main role of Th2 cells is to activate the humoral immune system as well as to secrete IL-4 and IL-5. IL-4 stimulates IgE production and IL-5 signals eosinophils **(Table 1)**. In pregnancy, the Th1/cytotoxic response is downregulated; whereas, the Th2 response predominates. Classically, immunoglobulin E (IgE) and eosinophils, through the Th2 pathway, are involved in the immune response against helminths (parasitic worms); whereas, cytotoxic T cells and macrophages, through the Th1 pathway, are recruited to a greater extent against protozoan infection. Thus, although helminthic infection can be dangerous in pregnancy, the severity of maternal, placental, and fetal infection is not as severe as with protozoan infections, which are generally managed by the cytotoxic immune system **(Table 1)**.

The maternal immune system may tolerate fetal antigens by suppressing cell-mediated immunity while retaining normal humoral immunity. These changes are known to occur locally at the maternal–fetal interface but may also affect systemic immune responses to infection. Although pregnant women are not immunosuppressed in the classic sense, immunologic changes in pregnancy may induce a state of increased susceptibility to certain intracellular pathogens, including viruses, intracellular bacteria, and parasites.

TABLE 1: General tenets of immune response to parasitic infections.

Helminthic	*Protozoa*
Th2 cells produce IL-4 and IL-5	Th1 cells produce IFN-γ
IL-4 and IL-5 stimulate the production of IgE	IFN-γ activates macrophages
IgE activates mast cells and eosinophils	Macrophage activation allows the destruction of intracellular parasites

(IFN-γ: interferon-gamma; IgE: immunoglobulin E; IL-4: interleukin 4; Th2: T-helper cell 2)

MATERNAL–FETAL INTERFACE

The fetal allograft is exposed to the maternal immune system at the placenta and fetal membranes (the amnion and chorion), collectively described as the maternal–fetal interface. On the fetal side of the interface, the placenta and membranes enclose the fetus and are derived entirely from fetal tissue. Forming a specialized epithelial surface within the placenta, fetal syncytiotrophoblast cells directly contact maternal blood for nutrient exchange. On the maternal side of the interface, the uterine tissue in contact with the placenta and fetal membranes, the decidua, is rich in specialized maternal immune cells including lymphocytes and macrophages.[2] Despite the prolonged direct exposure of decidual leukocytes and maternal blood to fetal antigens, the immune system does not recognize the fetus as foreign. Several mechanisms underlie this maternal tolerance of fetal tissues.

HUMORAL IMMUNITY

Humoral immunity is also known as antibody-mediated immunity. Humoral immunity results from the recognition of pathogens by specific antibodies. Most effective against extracellular pathogens, humoral immunity is essential for fighting many bacterial infections. The bacteria become coated in antibodies, which then mediate the uptake of the pathogens by phagocytic cells, including neutrophils and macrophages. The presentation of the bacterial antigens on the surface of the macrophage then stimulates B lymphocytes specific to the pathogen, and the B cells produce more antibodies to control the infection. This humoral immune response is augmented by Th2 lymphocytes, which provide costimulation and induce replication of the B-cells. The Th2 response during pregnancy results in vigorous antibody-mediated immunity to pathogens.[2]

CELL-MEDIATED IMMUNITY

Essential for controlling intracellular pathogens, cell-mediated immunity involves lymphocyte recognition of cell-associated foreign antigens, followed by destruction of the infected host cells. In contrast to humoral immunity, this arm of the immune response is stimulated by T-helper type I (Th1) lymphocytes and the cytokines they release. The most important effectors of the cell-mediated immune response, cytotoxic T lymphocytes, are the main immune cells that recognize foreign antigens on the surface of infected "self" cells. Cells infected with viruses or other intracellular pathogens are cytotoxic T lymphocytes' most common targets. The cell-mediated immune response is critical for controlling such pathogens because their intracellular location shelters them from antibody binding.

T-HELPER CELLS AND THE TH1-TH2 SHIFT

Emphasis on cell-mediated immunity versus humoral immunity changes according to the type of T-helper lymphocytes responding to an infectious threat. Multiple factors, including the cytokine environment and costimulatory molecules present during activation of the T-helper cell, determine the development of either Th1- or Th2-helper phenotype. One hypothesis is that, in addition to hormonal factors that affect the Th1-Th2 balance, macrophages present at the maternal–fetal interface release predominantly Th2-stimulating cytokines and contribute to the overall dominance of humoral immunity during pregnancy.[3] In addition to stimulating B lymphocytes, Th2 cells suppress the cytotoxic T lymphocyte response, decreasing the robustness of cell-mediated immunity. Recent studies show that progesterone binds to a blocking factor induced by the same hormone (PBF) in T lymphocytes. This binding induces the grouping of JAK homodimers, which triggers the activation of the STAT6 pathway. Once STAT6 is activated, it is translocated to the nucleus, thus promoting transcription of IL-4, IL-10, and TGF-β. These cytokines, in turn, inhibit the Th1 response and promote the Th2 response, a mechanism that prompts the generation of immunoglobulins **(Fig. 1)**. This is the mechanism by which progesterone can inhibit the Th1 type response and exacerbate the Th2 type response, characterized by increased IL-4, IL-5, and IL-10 levels. In the uterine decidua, the Th2 cytokine environment favors the activation of B lymphocytes, resulting in the stimulation of antibody secretion and suppression of cell-mediated immunity.[3] This phenomenon is often referred to as the Th1-Th2 shift of pregnancy and is thought to contribute to maternal tolerance of the fetus by suppressing the antifetal cell-mediated immune response. However, this type of immunity may entail higher susceptibility towards Th1-dependent parasitic infections, like those caused by Leishmania major. These infections not only present an increase in Th2 type immunity but also a decrease in Th1 type immunity. In infections caused by *Neospora caninum* and *Toxoplasma gondii*, the number of parasites correlates with the decrease in IL-2 and INF-γ (Th1 type immunity), while the Th2 type has no effect on infection.

SYSTEMIC IMMUNE CHANGES

An evolving model of pregnancy-associated immune changes suggests that the hormonal environment of pregnancy contributes to local suppression of cell-mediated immunity at the maternal–fetal interface while mediating a systemic change toward Th2 dominance. The fact that the local Th1–Th2 shift may also influence the systemic maternal immune response during pregnancy is evidenced in pregnant patients with autoimmune disorders. Women with rheumatoid arthritis, a predominantly cell-mediated autoimmune disorder, tend to experience remissions during pregnancy.[4]

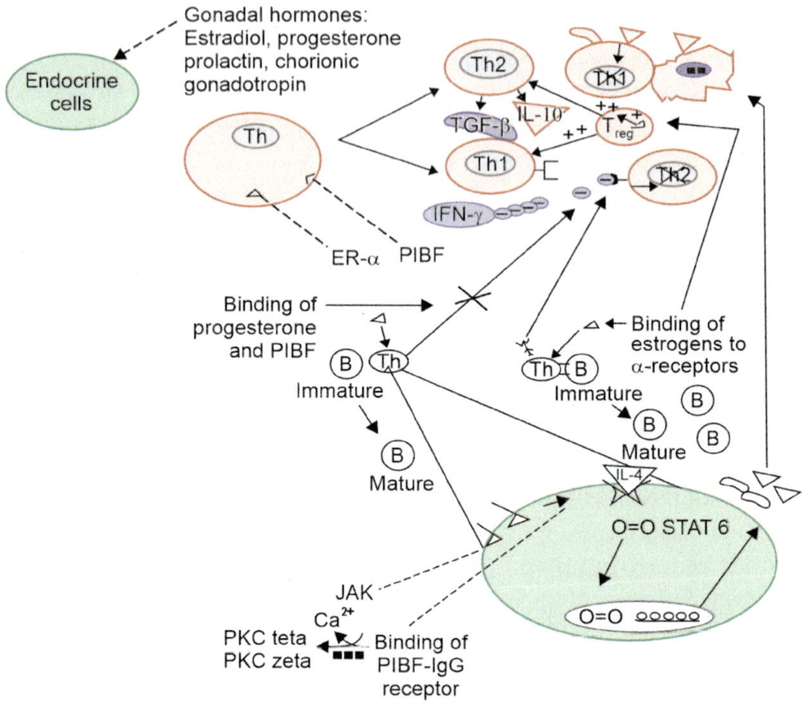

Fig. 1: Cellular communication among the different systems. Mode of interaction of progesterone and estradiol with T lymphocyte through the protein PIBF. Once it binds to the receptor, phosphorylation ensues by which the JAK/STAT6 receptors are activated, inducing transcription of IL-4, IL-10, and TGF-β. These cytokines and T_{reg} production inhibit Th1 and promote the Th2 type response.[7] (IL: interleukin; PIBF: progesterone-induced blocking factor; STAT6: signal transducer and activator of transcription 6; TGF-β: Transforming growth factor beta; Th2: T-helper cell type 2)
Source: Vargas-Villavicencio JA, De León-Nava MA, Morales-Montor J. Immunoendocrine Mechanisms Associated with Resistance or Susceptibility to Parasitic Diseases during Pregnancy. Neuroimmunomodulation. 2009;16(2):114-21.

Similarly, patients with multiple sclerosis have fewer exacerbations while pregnant but worsening symptoms during the postpartum period.[5] Systemic lupus erythematosus, however, a predominantly antibody-mediated autoimmune disorder, often worsens during pregnancy, perhaps due to increased immunoglobulin synthesis and decreased clearance of immune complexes resulting from robust Th2 activity.[3,6] These well-studied changes in the severity of autoimmune disorders during pregnancy illustrate systemic immune alterations that occur in conjunction with the Th1–Th2 shift. Systemic suppression of cell-mediated immunity may contribute to increased susceptibility to some intracellular pathogens including viruses, bacteria, and parasites during pregnancy.

REFERENCES

1. Adams K, Shields L. Maternal-fetal immunology. In: Gabbe SG, Niebyl JR, Simpson JL (Eds). Obstetrics: Normal and Problem Pregnancies, 5th edition. Philadelphia, PA: Churchill Livingstone; 2007. pp. 85-101.
2. Gaunt G, Ramin K. Immunological tolerance of the human fetus. Am J Perinatol. 2001;18(6):299-312.
3. Szekeres-Bartho J. Immunological relationship between the mother and the fetus. Int Rev Immunol. 2002;21(6):471-95.
4. Elenkov IJ, Wilder RL, Bakalov VK, Link AA, Dimitrov MA, Fisher S, et al. IL-12, TNF-alpha, and hormonal changes during late pregnancy and early postpartum: implications for autoimmune disease activity during these times. J Clin Endocrinol Metab. 2001;86(10):4933-8.
5. Runmarker B, Andersen O. Pregnancy is associated with a lower risk of onset and a better prognosis in multiple sclerosis. Brain. 1995;118(Pt 1):253-61.
6. Imrie HJ, McGonigle TP, Liu DT, Jones DR. Reduction in erythrocyte complement receptor 1 (CR1, CD35) and decay accelerating factor (DAF, CD55) during normal pregnancy. J Reprod Immunol. 1996;31(3):221-7.
7. Vargas-Villavicencio JA, De León-Nava MA, Morales-Montor J. Immunoendocrine Mechanisms Associated with Resistance or Susceptibility to Parasitic Diseases during Pregnancy. Neuroimmunomodulation. 2009;16(2):114-21.

CHAPTER 4

Malaria in Pregnancy

INTRODUCTION

Malaria is one of the most prevalent parasitic infestations in the world. It is endemic to most of the tropical countries of Asia, South America, and Africa. In pregnancy, it could present as a cause of severe hemolytic anemia and periodic fever episodes. Due to the high endemicity of the disease in India, it is important to rule out malaria in pregnant women with fever and anemia. Prophylaxis and treatment of this disease are widely available and therefore it is important to be aware of the presentation, diagnosis, complications, and management.

PATHOPHYSIOLOGY

Malaria is caused by infection with an obligate intracellular protozoan of the genus Plasmodium. Four main species are known to infect humans.

These are:

- *Plasmodium falciparum*
- *Plasmodium vivax*
- *Plasmodium malariae*
- *Plasmodium ovale*

After the bite of a female anopheline mosquito, the erythrocyte is infected with the sporozoites of the protozoan. In a few minutes, the sporozoites invade the hepatocytes and undergo asexual multiplication to for merozoites. This is the exoerythrocytic phase. During this phase, there may be no symptoms. Once the hepatocyte undergoes rupture, the merozoites are released into the bloodstream and again invade the erythrocytes. In 48–72 hours after invasion of the erythrocyte, trophozoites and subsequently schizonts with daughter merozoites are formed. The erythrocyte will rupture and the released daughter merozoites infect other erythrocytes. Thus, the erythrocytic phase continues. Few of the merozoites undergo sexual maturation to form gametocytes. These gametocytes are infective to anopheline mosquitos. Upon ingestion of the gametocyte, it undergoes maturation in the stomach of the mosquito and further migrates to the salivary gland of the mosquito. This is how the transmission occurs through the mosquitos. **Figure 1** shows the life cycle of a malarial parasite.

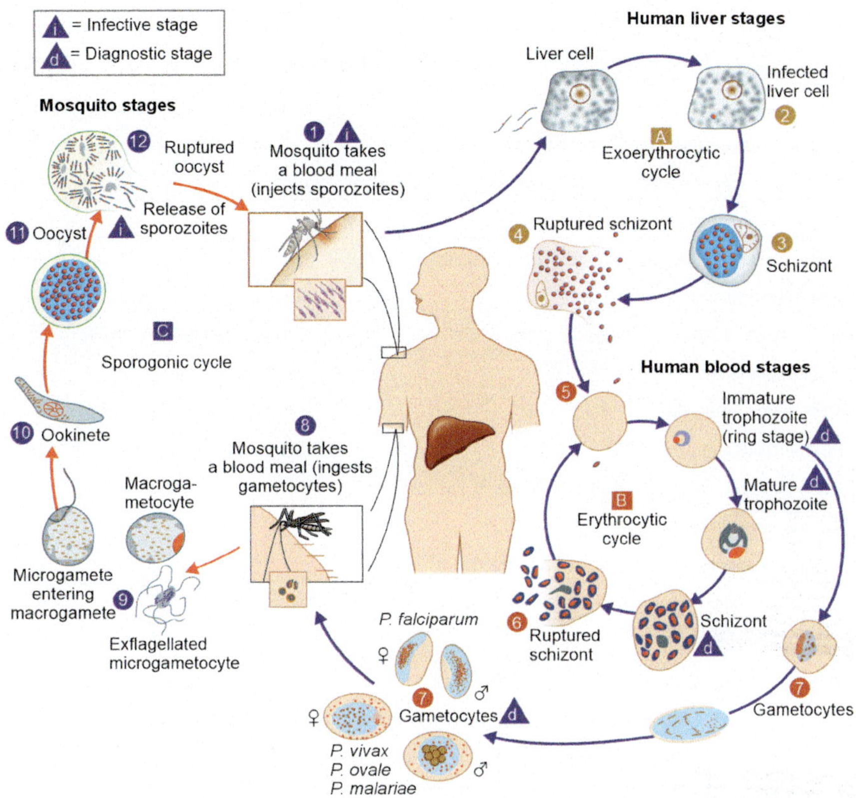

Fig. 1: Life cycle of the malaria parasite.
Source: National Center for Emerging and Zoonotic Infectious Diseases (NCEZID). Division of Parasitic Diseases and Malaria. [Online] Available from https://www.cdc.gov/ncezid/divisions-offices/about-dpdm.html [Last accessed November, 2024].

Other modes of transmission are:
- Through blood transfusion
- Congenital malaria

In these modes of transmission, there is no exoerythrocytic phase. Therefore, relapses are uncommon and also long-term treatment to eradicate hepatic form is unnecessary.

MATERNAL INFECTION

The host immunity and the infecting parasite play a role in deciding the severity of infection. Of particular concern in India is the fact that pregnancy is associated with a significant fall in immunity levels due to which the is a greater degree of parasitemia and clinical symptoms.

The symptoms are variable, most commonly:
- Chills

TABLE 1: Fever periodicity in malaria.

Organism	*Fever periodicity*
Plasmodium falciparum	Every 24–48 hours
Plasmodium vivax and *Plasmodium ovale*	Every 48 hours (alternate day)
Plasmodium malariae	Every 72 hours

TABLE 2: Features of malaria in pregnancy.

Nonobstetric	*Obstetric*
Fever with rigors	Mid trimester abortions
Hypersplenism	Premature labor
Hemolytic anemia	Fetal growth restriction
Folate deficiency	Intrapartum asphyxia
Convulsions (may be a feature of cerebral malaria)	Intrauterine fetal demise
Acute renal insufficiency	
Disseminated intravascular coagulation	

- Fever
- Headache
- Myalgia

Paroxysms of fever are characterized by rigor episodes followed by a febrile period of approximately 6 hours **(Table 1)**.

One of the main features of malaria in pregnancy is the exaggeration of anemia of pregnancy. A strong clinical suspicion should be had if there is a combination of fever, hypersplenism, and evidence of hemolytic anemia. Folic acid deficiency can be precipitated due to high turnover of red blood cells. Lymphadenopathy is characteristically absent.

Placental insufficiency can cause second-trimester abortions, fetal growth restriction, intrauterine demise, fresh stillbirth due to intrapartum asphyxia, and premature labor. **Table 2** shows the features of malaria in pregnancy.

CONGENITAL MALARIA

The transmission of the parasite through the placenta depends on maternal immune status. There is a 30% incidence of placental malaria among women in endemic areas; however, only 10% of them are symptomatic for malaria.[1] Demonstration of parasites in the placenta is considered more accurate than maternal blood sampling for detecting fetal affection. Direct transmission of the parasite or transmission of Immunoglobulin G (IgG) from the maternal circulation is the postulated mechanism for the transmission of malaria in utero. Clinical features in the fetus may appear 2–4 weeks after birth and include fever, lethargy, anorexia, and in some cases convulsions.

Hepatosplenomegaly may be absent in the initial stages but develop rather quickly once the clinical features appear.[2]

DIAGNOSIS

It is based on clinical suspicion and demonstration of the parasite on thick and thin blood smears. If the smears are taken during the febrile paroxysms, the chances of obtaining the parasite are higher as this is the time when the schizonts burst and merozoites are released into the circulation. Giemsa stain is used to identify the species of the parasite which will then direct the treatment required. Nowadays, rapid diagnostic kits are available for the diagnosis of malaria.

MANAGEMENT IN PREGNANCY[3]

For prevention, a three-pronged strategy is recommended by the World Health Organization (WHO) in endemic areas, such as Africa. This includes:

1. Case management (using highly effective drugs and initiating the treatment promptly)
2. Prevention with insecticide-treated bed nets.
3. *Intermittent preventive treatment in pregnancy (IPTp)*: Administration of full course antimalarial treatment at regular antenatal visits. Sulfadoxine–pyrimethamine (SP) is generally used.

However, there is a lack of evidence regarding the benefit of IPTp in India. Also, there is low efficacy of SP against *P. vivax*, and low levels of uptake.

Thus, the treatment protocols differ based on the severity of infection and the species of implicated parasite.

Uncomplicated Falciparum Malaria

All children and adults (except pregnant women in the first trimester) should be treated with artemisinin-based combination therapy (ACT). ACT should provide at least 3 days of coverage with artemisinin derivative.

The combinations available are:

- Artemether + lumefantrine
- Artesunate + amodiaquine
- Artesunate + mefloquine
- Dihydroartemisinin + piperaquine
- Artesunate + sulfadoxine–pyrimethamine

These are available as Fixed dose combinations for various weight ranges. **Table 3** discusses the dosing of artemether and lumefantrine according to weight bands.

Table 4 highlights the dosing of artesunate + amodiaquine according to weight bands.

Tables 5 and 6 highlight the weight-wise dosage of artesunate + mefloquine and artesunate + sulfadoxine/pyrimethamine, respectively.

TABLE 3: Dosing of artemether + lumefantrine.

Artemether + lumefantrine (twice daily for 3 days).	
Body weight (kg)	***Dose (mg) (Am +Lf)***
5 to <15	20 + 120
15 to <25	40 + 240
25 to <35	60 + 360
≥35	80 + 480

Note:
- Lumefantrine exposure is known to be decreased in pregnant women. Thus, treatment response should be closely monitored in them.
- This artemisinin-based combination therapy (ACT) is preferred because lumefantrine is not available as a monotherapy, hence incidence of resistance is less.
- Lumefantrine is better absorbed along with fat. Hence, patients are to be instructed to take the tablets along with milk after a full meal.

TABLE 4: Dosing of artesunate + amodiaquine.

Artesunate + Amodiaquine (daily for 3 days)	
Body weight (kg)	***Dose (mg) (As +Aq)***
4.5 to <9	25 + 67.5
9 to <18	50 + 135
18 to <36	100 + 270
>36	540

Note: There is no significant change in the pharmacokinetics of amodiaquine in pregnancy. Hence, dose adjustment is not required.

TABLE 5: Dosing of artesunate + mefloquine.

Artesunate + mefloquine (daily for 3 days)	
Body weight (kg)	***Dose (mg) (As +Aq)***
5 to <9	25 + 55
9 to <18	50 + 110
18 to <30	100 + 220
≥30	200 + 440

Uncomplicated Falciparum Malaria in the First Trimester of Pregnancy

The commonly used regimen for uncomplicated *P. falciparum* malaria in the first trimester of pregnancy is 7 days of quinine + clindamycin (10 mg/kg body weight).

TABLE 6: Dosing of artesunate + sulfadoxine/pyrimethamine

Body weight (kg)	*Artesunate dose (mg) (daily for 3 days)*	*Sulfadoxine + pyrimethamine dose (mg) (single dose on day 1)*
5 to <10	25	250 + 12.5
10 to <25	50	500 + 25
25 to <50	100	1,000 + 50
≥50	200	1,500 + 75

Note:
- This ACT is not available as a fixed dose combination.
- Thus, there is a risk of loose distribution of Artesunate tablets and treatment failures. Artesunate monotherapy is banned by the WHO.
- In areas with high endemicity, there is likely a high prevalence of sulfadoxine–pyrimethamine resistance.

(ACT: artemisinin-based combination therapy; WHO: World Health Organization)

Dosages in Lactation

Pharmacokinetics of most of the antimalarial drugs are not significantly altered in lactation. Tetracycline is contraindicated during lactation due to the potential adverse effects on the infant's bones and teeth. Primaquine should not be given during breastfeeding unless the breastfed infant has been checked for glucose-6-phosphate dehydrogenase deficiency (G6PD).

Uncomplicated *Plasmodium vivax, Plasmodium ovale* and *Plasmodium malariae* Infections

The main objective of treatment is to target both the erythrocytic stage as well as the hepatic stage of the parasite, known as *radical cure*.

- If the species is not known with certainty, treat it as uncomplicated falciparum malaria.
- In areas with chloroquine-sensitive malaria, treat uncomplicated *P. vivax, P. ovale,* and *P. malariae* infections with either ACT (except in the first trimester of pregnancy) or chloroquine (preferred in the first trimester of pregnancy).
- *Dose of chloroquine*: 10 mg base/kg body weight on day 1 and day 2, followed by 5 mg base/kg body weight on day 3 of treatment.
- In areas with chloroquine-resistant malaria, treat uncomplicated *P. vivax, P. ovale,* and *P. malariae* infections in the first trimester with quinine.
- *For preventing relapses*:
    - Weekly chemoprophylaxis with chloroquine can be considered till delivery or breastfeeding is completed.
    - Primaquine may be used only in women who are breastfeeding infants older than 6 months old, after documenting that the infant is not G6PD deficient.

SEVERE MALARIA DURING PREGNANCY

Second- and third-trimester pregnant women are more likely to have severe malaria compared to other adults. Pulmonary edema and hypoglycemia may complicate these cases. Intrauterine fetal demises and preterm labor are often seen. Maternal mortality with severe malaria is in the range of 50%.

Parenteral Artesunate in full dose should be immediately started. If artesunate is not available, Artemether intramuscular (IM) can be given. If this is also not available, treatment may be started with quinine till Artesunate is made available.

Severe *vivax* malaria may present with anemia, thrombocytopenia, pulmonary edema, cerebral malaria, pancytopenia, jaundice, splenic rupture, acute kidney injury, and shock. All these need to be concomitantly treated along with achieving radical cure through parenteral antimalarials.

CONCLUSION

Malaria is a common, mostly benign, and frequently underdiagnosed condition in pregnancy.

Simple combination therapies are available that help to achieve a complete cure and prevent maternal and perinatal morbidity and mortality.

Adherence to treatment, monitoring of clinical response, and high suspicion of drug resistance are imperative to avoid complications, relapse, and recrudescence.

REFERENCES

1. Larkin GL, Thuma PE. Congenital malaria in a hyperendemic area. Am J Trop Med Hyg. 1991;45(5):587-92.
2. Nyirjesy P, Kavasy T, Axelrod P, Fisher PR. Malaria during pregnancy: Neonatal morbidity and mortality and the efficacy of chloroquine chemoprophylaxis. Clin Infect Dis. 1993;16(1):127-32.
3. World Health Organization. Guidelines for the treatment of malaria. Geneva: World Health Organization; 2015.

5 CHAPTER

Intestinal Infections in Pregnancy

ENTAMOEBA HISTOLYTICA

INTRODUCTION

The intestinal protozoan *Entamoeba histolytica* infects around 10% of the world's population.[1] Ileum and colon are the parasite's primary habitats. Despite the fact that amebiasis is typically seen as an asymptomatic carrier condition, *E. histolytica* can develop a variety of symptoms ranging from chronic mild diarrhea to fulminant dysentery. Extraintestinal problems, such as hepatic abscess, can also occur.

Figure 1 shows an electron microscopic image of *Entamoeba histolytica*.

ORGANISM AND ITS TRANSMISSION

There are several *Entamoeba* species that can infect humans, although not all of them are linked to disease. Among the several ameba species that normally parasitize the human mouth and gut, only *E. histolytica* has been related to gastrointestinal (GIT) disorders. *E. histolytica* is found as a motile trophozoite, precyst, or cyst. The trophozoite resides in the intestinal

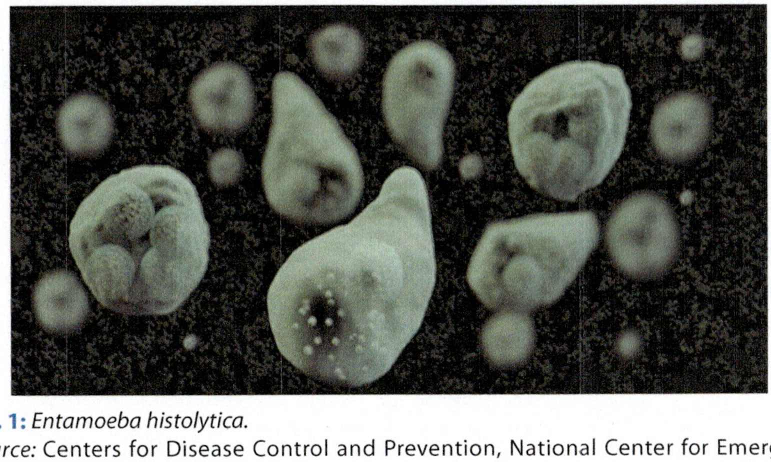

Fig. 1: *Entamoeba histolytica.*
Source: Centers for Disease Control and Prevention, National Center for Emerging and Zoonotic Infectious Diseases (NCEZID). Division of Foodborne, Waterborne, and Environmental Diseases. [Online] Available from: https://www.cdc.gov/ncezid/divisions-offices/about-dfwed.html [Last accessed November, 2024].

lumen and divides by binary fission; in the case of rapid transit, it may pass through liquid stool unaltered. It favors anaerobic environments and feeds on bacteria or tissue substrates to meet its nutritional needs. It has a nucleus and cytoplasm. Cytoplasm is divided into two types: (1) Clear ectoplasm and (2) Granular endoplasm. Trophozoites are actively motile with the help of pseudopodia. The trophozoite will normally encyst and pass in the stool if there is no diarrhea.

- *Precyst:* It is the intermediate stage between trophozoite and cyst which is smaller in size, round, or slightly ovoid in shape with blunt pseudopodium projecting from the periphery.
- Cysts, being the infective form of parasite with round or oval shape are quadrinucleate and contain glycogen vacuoles and chromatid bars. Cysts are extremely resistant to environmental changes, chlorine concentrations seen in water purification systems, and gastric acid in general.

Ingestion of cyst forms caused by fecal contamination of food or water is the most common way for the disease to spread. A cyst is resistant to gastric acid and therefore undergoes excystation in the cecum or ilium at neutral pH with the help of trypsin. Excystation gives rise to eight trophozoites which pass down to the large intestine, divide by binary fission, and attach to intestinal mucosa with the help of lectin, secretes proteolytic enzymes, and causes tissue necrosis. When they gain access to the bloodstream, it causes extraintestinal disease. When environmental conditions become unsuitable for continuing trophozoite proliferation, these organisms encyst. **Figure 2** explains the life cycle of *E. histolytica.*

EPIDEMIOLOGY

The prevalence of *E. histolytica* varies according to the community's cleanliness and personal hygiene.[2,3] In tropical places with poor sanitation, rates may reach 50–80%. The overall prevalence in the United States is estimated to be between 3 and 5%, although, in institutions for the intellectually disabled, homosexual male communities, and migrant labor camps, it may reach around 40%.

CLINICAL MANIFESTATIONS

Intestinal Amebiasis

Colonic irritation, characterized by colicky lower stomach pain with or without diarrhea, is the most prevalent symptom of an amebic disease. The stool is loose, foul-smelling, large, and brownish-black often streaked with blood or mucus. On physical examination, the abdomen may be tender. Pregnant women are more likely to have acute flare-ups of amebic disease and more visible symptoms.[4,5] Bloody, dysenteric stools, moderate abdominal pain, and tenderness are common clinical manifestations in

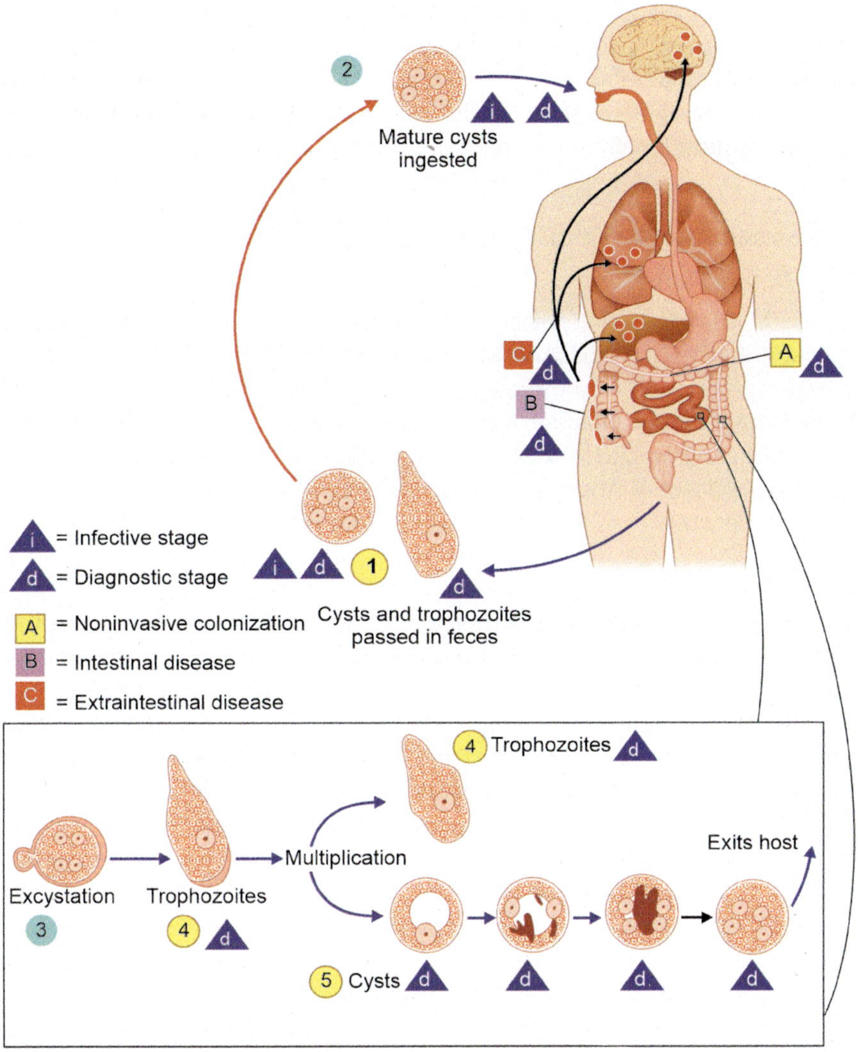

Fig. 2: Life cycle of *Entamoeba histolytica*.
Source: Centers for Disease Control and Prevention, National Center for Emerging and Zoonotic Infectious Diseases (NCEZID), Division of Foodborne, Waterborne, and Environmental Diseases (DFWED). Life cycle of Entamoeba histolytica. [Online] Available from: https://www.cdc.gov/dpdx/amebiasis/modules/Amebiasis_LifeCycle_lg.jpg [Last accessed November, 2024].

pregnant women who are infected. As a result of the severe diarrhea, fluid loss, and electrolyte imbalance could have a detrimental effect on the pregnancy's outcome.[6] Neither the placenta nor the fetus have been shown to be infected by the parasite. Pregnancy or the use of corticosteroids can cause amebic dysentery to become fulminant.[7] Rectosigmoid ulceration can be seen on sigmoidoscopy and rarely colonic mucosal destruction with bowel perforation and hemorrhage may be seen. The radiological diagnosis of an ameboma in the cecum, which is rare can be mistaken for that of adenocarcinoma. Complications such as toxic megacolon, fulminant amoebic colitis, ameboma, amoebic peritonitis, and perianal ulceration may occur.

Extraintestinal Amebiasis

Hepatic Infection

When *E. histolytica* migrates to the liver, it can cause an abscess or nonsuppurative hepatitis. Amebiasis in pregnancy does not appear to cause hepatic amebiasis. Hepatic abscess occurs more frequently in cases of asymptomatic colon infection than in those of symptomatic colonic infection. Fever, sweating, weight loss, and painful hepatomegaly are all symptoms of a developing abscess. Abscess is frequently seen in the right lobe of the liver, and it is most commonly found in the posterior portion of the right lobe.

Pulmonary Infection

A hepatic abscess can extend upward, rupture through the diaphragm, and may cause pleural effusions and pulmonary infection causing pulmonary abscess. It may cause chest pain, dyspnea, or nonproductive cough.

Hepatic amebiasis can also cause rupture into the pericardium and peritoneum, which is a more dangerous consequence. Depending on the site of rupture, the clinical signs are those of a moribund patient with evidence of pleural effusion, pericardial tamponade, or acute abdomen.

Cerebral Infection

Brain abscesses can also develop as a complication of hepatic abscess and may present as seizures or coma.

Other complications include genitourinary amoebiasis, splenic infection, or cutaneous amoebiasis.

DIAGNOSIS

Sample for diagnosis includes stool, pus of a liver abscess, sputum, and biopsy sample.

Stool Examination

- Macroscopically, stools are foul smelling, semi-solid in consistency, dark brown in color, mixed with blood or mucus.
- Microscopically, motile trophozoites with red blood cells (RBCs) in their cytoplasm can be examined in saline wet mount preparation of stool. Charcot-Leyden crystals can be seen. Multiple stool examinations are necessary due to the variable excretion of cysts and trophozoites.

For the detection of cysts, stools are to be fixed in polyvinyl alcohol (PVA) or formalin and concentrated in formalin-ether.
- Stool antigen detection by enzyme-linked immunosorbent assay (ELISA).
- Stool culture in Robinson's medium and NH polyxenic culture medium.

Extraintestinal amoebiasis:
- *Serology:* To detect antibodies in serum against *E. histolytica*. Enzyme immunoassay kits for antibody detection have a specificity of 95% for extraintestinal amoebiasis, 70% for intestinal amoebiasis, and 10% for asymptomatic carriers. If an antibody is detected in a dilution of ≥1:128, the indirect hemagglutination test (IHA) is considered positive.
- *Radiology:* Amebic abscess is diagnosed via radioisotopic scanning, computed tomography, and ultrasonography of the liver which appears as a solitary defect in the right lobe. Chest X-ray (CXR) to rule out pulmonary involvement.
- *Microscopy:* An odorless, brownish "anchovy paste" liquid is aspirated from a liver abscess which may contain trophozoites. Amoebae are usually confined to the periphery of an abscess.

TREATMENT

Amebiasis treatment should focus on symptomatic management such as fluid and electrolyte imbalance, blood transfusion if required, and pathogen elimination. Drug therapy for amoebiasis in pregnancy should be administered according to the severity of the disease as many antiparasitic drugs are contraindicated during pregnancy.

Treatment for asymptomatic carrier pregnant women is to be postponed beyond 14 weeks of pregnancy or after birth. A drug used is metronidazole 750 mg TDS PO for 5–7 days.[8] Paromomycin 30 mg/kg/day in three divided doses for seven days can be a safe alternative.

Metronidazole for 10 days is the preferred treatment for extraintestinal amebiasis, including hepatic abscess. The most successful treatment in bowel perforation or peritonitis is to keep the peritoneum draining whilst using adequate antibiotics.

GIARDIA LAMBLIA INFECTION

In the United States, *G. lamblia* is the most common protozoan that causes diarrhea in travelers and waterborne outbreaks. *G. lamblia* is also known as *Giardia intestinalis* or *Giardia duodenalis*.

Giardiasis, such as amebiasis, is present all over the world, with a global incidence of 7%.

Giardiasis is characterized by persistent diarrhea and malabsorption, and it is most commonly encountered in communities with poor sanitation and people with poor personal hygiene.[9]

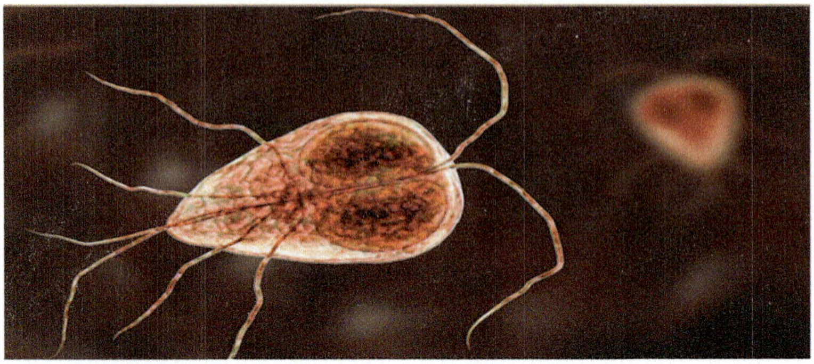

Fig. 3: *Giardia lamblia.*
Source: Centers for Disease Control and Prevention, National Center for Emerging and Zoonotic Infectious Diseases (NCEZID), Division of Foodborne, Waterborne, and Environmental Diseases (DFWED). Life cycle of Entamoeba histolytica. [Online] Available from: https://www.cdc.gov/dpdx/amebiasis/modules/Amebiasis_LifeCycle_lg.jpg [Last accessed November, 2024].

ORGANISM AND ITS TRANSMISSION

Giardia lamblia is a multiflagellated protozoan that exists in two morphological forms: (1) Trophozoite and cyst. **Figure 3** shows the structure of *G. lamblia.*

Trophozoites are pear-shaped and measure 12–15 μm in length and 5–7 μm in width with two median bodies, two nuclei without nucleoli, four pairs of flagella, and a ventral sucking disc. The organism's two nuclei and central parabasal body give it the appearance of a face with two huge eyes when viewed under a microscope.

In humans, infection begins with ingestion of the cyst form from contaminated hands, water, or food. Excystation occurs in the acidic environment of the stomach and duodenum. With the alkaline pH being favorable, trophozoites remain in the duodenum and upper jejunum.

Giardia trophozoites multiply by longitudinal or binary fission and then adhere to the enterocytes by ventral sucking disc. Some trophozoites pass down to the colon and encyst in the presence of neutral pH and bile salts and these cysts after maturation are excreted in the feces. A cyst is oval or ellipsoidal in shape measuring 8–12 μm in length and has a thick cyst wall, granulated cytoplasm, and four nuclei. They can survive for months in cold water. Ingestion of contaminated water containing Giardia cysts acts as a source of infection. **Figure 4** shows the life cycle of *G. lamblia.*

EPIDEMIOLOGY

Giardiasis is widespread throughout the world, with a predominance in places with inadequate sanitation. In developed countries, the incidence is 2–5%, but in developing countries, it is 20–30%. It affects children three times

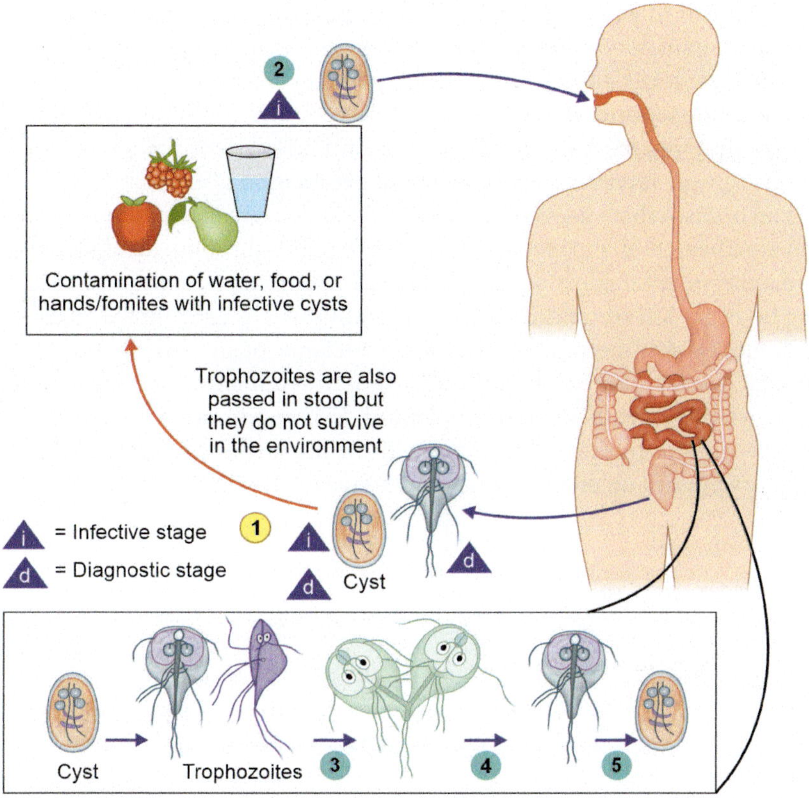

Fig. 4: Life cycle of *Giardia lamblia*.
Source: Global Health, Division of Parasitic Diseases and Malaria. Parasitic Diseases and Malaria. [Online] Available from https://www.cdc.gov/dpdx/giardiasis/index.html [Last accessed November, 2024].

more than adults and has more clinical symptoms. Adults with gastrectomy, lower gastric acidity, and chronic pancreatitis may be more susceptible. A lack of intestinal immunoglobulin A has been linked to giardiasis.

Routes of transmission:[10]

- *Feco-oral*:
  - Ingestion of contaminated water—most important
  - Ingestion of contaminated food
- Person-to-person—daycare, nursing homes, mental asylums (poor hygiene)[13]
- Sexual—sexually active homosexual males

CLINICAL MANIFESTATIONS

Symptoms vary widely in patients infected with *G. lamblia* from asymptomatic carriage to severe diarrhea and malabsorption. Symptomatic disease usually occurs after an incubation period of 1–2 weeks and is characterized by the sudden onset of watery diarrhea, abdominal distension, abdominal pain, flatulence, nausea, vomiting, and anorexia and usually lasts for 1–3 weeks. Occasionally fever and constipation may occur. Feces are frequently foul-smelling, loose, and mucus-laden. If not treated in some patients, the disease may progress to chronic infection and present with steatorrhea, malabsorption, recurrent symptoms, and debilitation.[14]

The unfavorable effects of *Giardia* infection on pregnancy are associated with diarrhea, fluid and electrolyte loss, and malabsorption, all of which can have a detrimental effect on the pregnancy's ultimate outcome.[11] Giardiasis may be more severe and resistant to treatment if a pregnant woman has dysgammaglobulinemia. Mechanical blockage of microvilli due to the physical barrier created by trophozoites between the intestinal lumen and enterocytes leads to inadequate absorption, enterocyte damage, villi atrophy, and crypt hyperplasia. Lectins present on the surface of giardia bind to receptors present on enterocytes and damage microvilli.[12]

DIAGNOSIS

Stool Examination

Microscopy

Because of the quick intestinal transit in the acute stage of the disease, feces are typically watery and loose and may contain trophozoites.

- On direct wet mount preparation, typical "falling leaf type" motility of trophozoite is seen.
- On iodine wet mount or trichrome stain, the cyst can be seen.
- *Concentration method:* Formalin-ether concentration or PVA is used for the concentration of stool and identification of the cyst with better parasite yield for microscopy. When stool exams consistently yield negative results, duodenal intubation with duodenal contents aspiration and duodenal biopsy may be used to confirm the diagnosis.
- *Microscopy with direct fluorescent antibody testing (DFA)*: The test of choice for diagnosis of giardia due to its increased sensitivity. Antibodies labeled with fluorescent markers are added to the stool sample and incubated. The giardia cysts appear as green, glowing ovoid objects when viewed under a fluorescent microscope. **Figure 5** shows cysts of *G. duodenalis* (lower right) and *Cryptosporidium* (upper left) labeled with commercially available immunofluorescent antibodies.
- Enzyme-linked immunosorbent assay for *Giardia* antigen in stool.
    - Stool culture
    - *Enterotest*: A gelatin capsule containing a nylon string with a weight attached to it is swallowed by the patient, with one end of a string attached to the cheek with the help of tape. The Gelatin capsule gets dissolved in the stomach, and the nylon string goes further down to

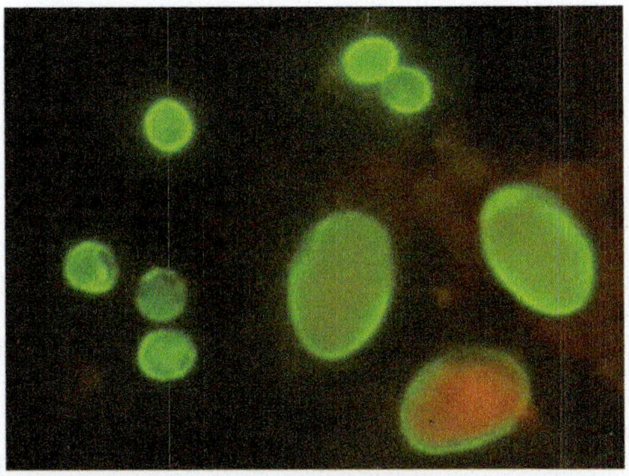

Fig. 5: Cysts of *Giardia duodenalis* (lower right) and *Cryptosporidium* (upper left) labeled with commercially available immunofluorescent antibodies.

Source:

1. Global Health, Division of Parasitic Diseases and Malaria. [Online] Available from: https://www.cdc.gov/dpdx/giardiasis/index.html [Last accessed November, 2024].
2. Global Health, Division of Parasitic Diseases and Malaria. [Online] Available from: https://www.cdc.gov/dpdx/giardiasis/images/7/Giardia_cyst_IFA.jpg [Last accessed November, 2024].

the duodenum and jejunum due to the attached weight. It is allowed to remain there for 4–6 hours after which the string is pulled back up and the contents are used as samples for examination.

TREATMENT

Pregnant women should receive therapy only if they are severely symptomatic because the infection may be self-limited in many persons. For pregnancy, a trial with paromomycin 10 mg/kg three times a day for 1 week is recommended. If symptoms persist or are severe, metronidazole may be used. Other drugs effective against *Giardia* include furazolidone and tinidazole.[11]

INFECTION WITH INTESTINAL NEMATODES

INTRODUCTION

Nematodes commonly affecting man are *Ascaris lumbricoides, Trichuris trichiura, Ancylostoma duodenale, Necator americanus, Strongyloides stercoralis,* and *Enterobius vermicularis*. These diseases are present worldwide and infect a large number of the population every year.[15]

ASCARIS LUMBRICOIDES

Organism and Its Life Cycle

The largest intestinal nematode or roundworm infects humans affecting >1 billion population worldwide. It is also one of the most common helminthic infections in men mainly affecting children between the ages of 2 and 10 years.

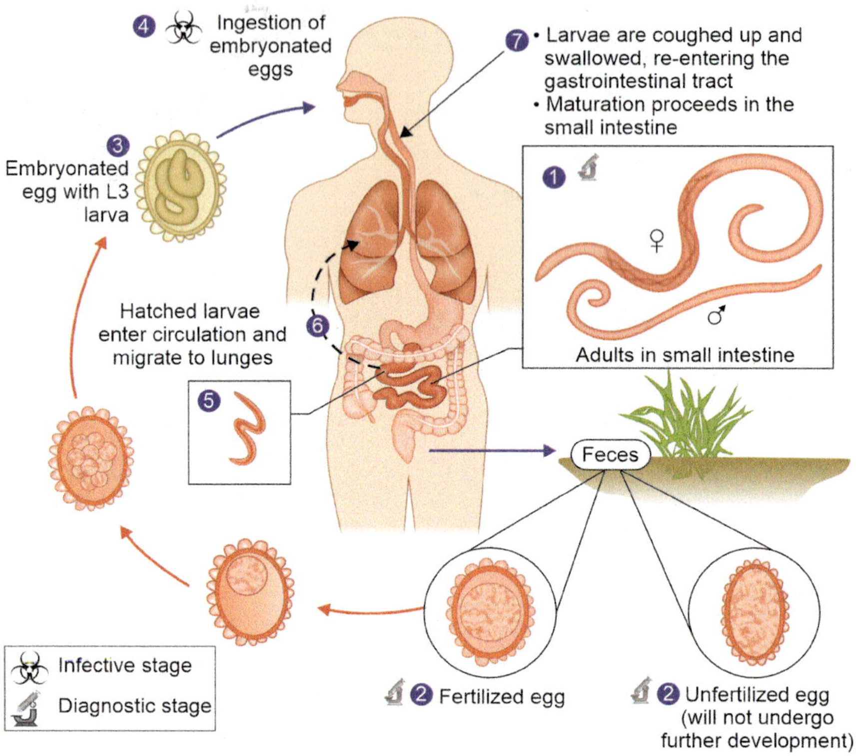

Fig. 6: Life cycle of *Ascaris lumbricoides*.
Source: CDC Global Health, Division of Parasitic Diseases and Malaria. [Online] Available from https://www.cdc.gov/parasites/ascariasis/biology.html [Last accessed November, 2024].

Humans acquire infection through ingestion of food or water contaminated with *Ascaris* embryonated eggs.[16] After ingestion, eggs release larvae in the duodenum from where they enter venous circulation, migrate to the lungs, enter the alveoli and grow there, ascend through the bronchial tree, and reach the trachea where they are coughed up and swallowed thus reaching the GIT tract again in the small intestine where they mature into adult worms.[17] Adult worms have a life span of 10–24 months. Female adult worms after fertilization produce around 2 lac fertilized eggs/day which pass in the feces and become infective after embryonation which takes around 18 days.[18] **Figure 6** shows the life cycle of *A. lumbricoides*.

Clinical Manifestations

Patients are usually asymptomatic, but symptoms are seen in individuals with high worm load. *Ascaris*, in patients who are not previously exposed to

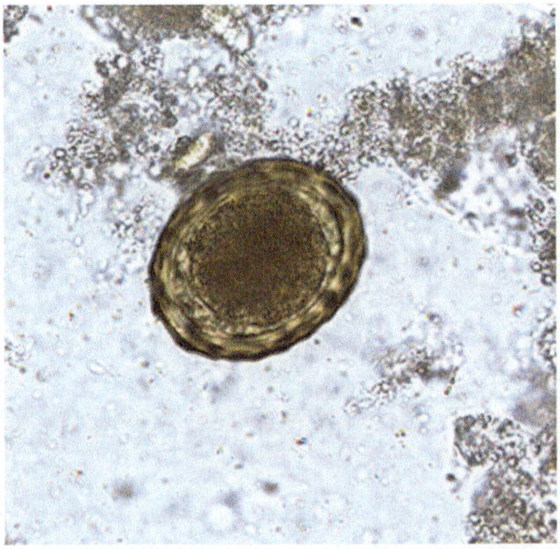

Fig. 7: Fertilized egg of *Ascaris lumbricoides* in an unstained wet mount of stool. *Source:* Global Health, Division of Parasitic Diseases and Malaria. DPDx. [Online] Available from https://www.cdc.gov/dpdx/ascariasis/images/2/Ascaris_fertile_BAM1.jpg [Last accessed November, 2024].

the worm, leads to Loeffler's syndrome which is a hypersensitivity reaction such as Katayama fever and manifests as fever, dry cough, dyspnea, wheeze, retrosternal discomfort, and hemoptysis and occurs during the migratory phase of larvae. On CXR, it is seen as a pulmonary infiltrate which is migratory, blood investigation shows eosinophilia and sputum examination shows Charcot-Leyden crystals.[24] During the late stages of infection, the intestinal phase, patients may complain of nausea, vomiting, abdominal pain, diarrhea, anorexia, and malnutrition.[20] If the worm burden is too high, it can cause intestinal obstruction, intussusception, appendicitis, and intestinal perforation.

Diagnosis and Treatment

Microscopy: Visualization of eggs in the feces is the mainstay for diagnosis owing to the large number of eggs excreted in feces.

Figure 7 shows the fertilized egg of *A. lumbricoides.* Pyrantel pamoate 11 mg/kg/day up to a maximum 1 g PO single dose. Alternatively, albendazole can be given in the second and third trimesters.

HOOKWORM

Organism and its Life Cycle

Around 500 million population in the world is infected with hookworm. Two major species infect man: (1) *A. duodenale* and (2) *N. americanus.* Organism resides in the small intestine and infection occurs predominantly in the

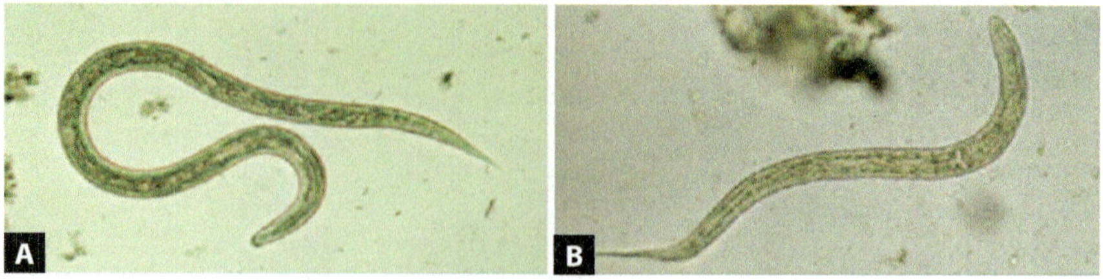

Figs. 8A and B: Left: *Filariform* (L3) hookworm larva in a wet mount. Right: Hookworm *rhabditiform* larva (wet preparation).
Source: CDC Global Health, Division of Parasitic Diseases and Malaria. Parasites. [Online] Available from https://www.cdc.gov/parasites/ [Last accessed November, 2024].

tropics and subtropics, such as sub-Saharan Africa, Asia, America, and the Caribbean.

Humans acquire infection by walking bare feet on contaminated soil where the larvae penetrate through the skin and cause infection. Larvae then gain access to the bloodstream, pass through the heart and reach the lungs, go into pulmonary alveoli and ascend up the bronchial tree to reach the trachea, get coughed up and swallowed thus finally reach the GIT tract. Larvae reach to small intestine in the jejunum, mature into adult worms, and reside in the jejunum for the rest of their life span of 1–2 years. **Figures 8A and B** show filariform and rhabditiform larvae. Female worms after fertilization lay around 7,000 eggs/day which gets excreted in the feces. These eggs hatch in the soil releasing rhabditiform larvae which further develop into filariform larvae. Filariform larvae are the infective form of the parasite which penetrates human skin.

Adult worms have a cylindrical body with a ventral buccal capsule through which it attaches to the intestine, consisting of six teeth, four hooks like on the ventral surface, and two knob-like on the dorsal surface.
Life cycle of intestinal hookworm is depicted in **Figure 9**.

Clinical Manifestations

A maculopapular pruritic rash appears at the site of entry of infective larvae on the skin typically called "ground itch." Sometimes serpiginous tract similar to cutaneous larva migrans may be seen. Migration of the larval form through the lungs may cause slight pharyngeal irritation and cough and sometimes hypersensitivity reaction may be seen. GIT symptoms such as nausea, vomiting, diarrhea, epigastric pain, and flatulence are some of the symptoms. With heavy infection, overt bleeding from GIT can be seen. Adult worm thrives on blood from host tissue thus hookworms lead to anemia due to loss of blood from the GIT (around 0.3–0.5 mL blood/day ingested by each worm). It also causes protein loss from the body. Hookworm infection in pregnant females can lead to low birth weight of babies owing to iron deficiency anemia, and hypoalbuminemia caused by worm infestation.

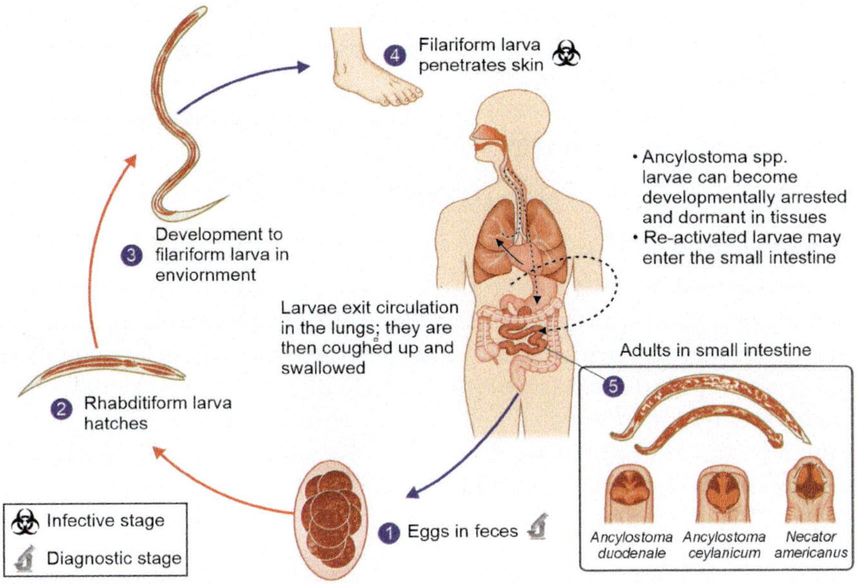

Fig. 9: Life cycle of intestinal hookworm.
Source: Global Health, Division of Parasitic Diseases and Malaria. Hookworm (Intestinal). [Online] Available from https://www.cdc.gov/dpdx/hookworm/index.html#tabs-2-3 [Last accessed November, 2024].

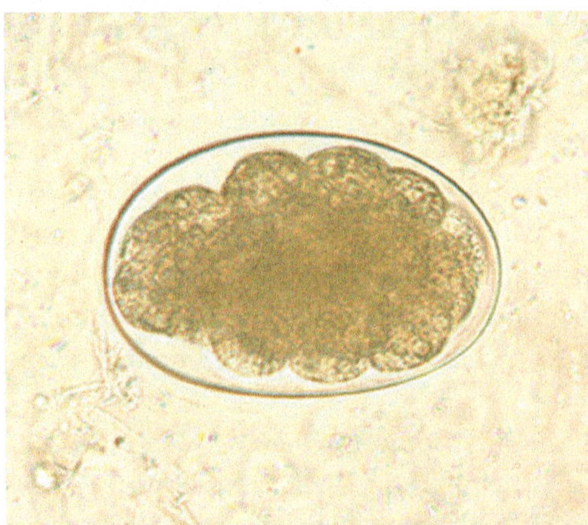

Fig. 10: Hookworm egg in an unstained wet mount, taken at 400× magnification.
Source: Global Health, Division of Parasitic Diseases and Malaria. [Online] Available from https://www.cdc.gov/dpdx/hookworm/images/1/Hookworm_egg_BAM1.jpg [Last accessed November, 2024].

Diagnosis and Treatment

Microscopy

Demonstration of eggs in feces may help in diagnosis. **Figure 10** demonstrates a hookworm egg under a microscope. Usually, diagnosis is established clinically with symptoms. Mebendazole at a dose of 100 mg BD PO for 3 days can be given to symptomatic pregnant women.[23] Alternatively, Pyrantel pamoate 11 mg/kg PO as a single dose can be used. Supportive therapy with iron supplementation, vitamins, and protein supplementation, or transfusion of blood and blood products if needed.[24]

STRONGYLOIDES STERCORALIS

Organism and its Life Cycle

Strongyloides stercoralis also known as dwarf threadworm, is the smallest nematode known to infect humans, with soil contaminated with human feces being the main source of infection. Parasites gain entry through penetration of the skin by filariform larvae with the help of proteolytic enzymes while walking barefoot in infected soil. These larvae then gain access to the bloodstream or lymphatics, migrate to the lungs, causing cough, get swallowed, and reach the small intestine where they mature into adult worms.[25] The female parasite resides in the tunnels between enterocytes of jejunal mucosa and produces eggs by parthenogenesis. Eggs hatch and produce rhabditiform larvae which may be excreted in stools or develop into filariform infective larvae. Rhabditiform larvae excreted in stools develop into free-living adult male and female worms which after fertilization produce eggs that hatch and form rhabditiform larvae which further develop into infective filariform larvae in the soil. The infectious filariform larvae may penetrate colonic or perianal skin areas and reinfect the host, thus known as "autoinfection." **Figure 11** shows the life cycle of *S. stercoralis*.

Clinical Manifestations

Maximum infected patients are asymptomatic.

- *Cutaneous symptoms*: Migration through the skin may produce a typical serpiginous urticarial rash called "larva currens" (racing larvae).[27] Erythema and itching may be present at the site of entry of larvae. Chronic strongyloidiasis presents as pruritus and urticarial in the perianal skin and buttocks.
- *Pulmonary symptoms*: Cough, wheezing, dyspnea, and hemoptysis may occur as a result of the migration of larvae in the lungs. Bronchopneumonia, chronic bronchitis, or asthma-like symptoms are seen in some patients.
- *Intestinal infection*: Abdominal pain, epigastric discomfort, nausea, vomiting, diarrhea, and tenderness may be present. Malabsorption or protein-losing enteropathy and paralytic ileus may be seen in some.[26]

Diagnosis and Treatment

Stool Examination

- *Microscopy*: Demonstration of rhabditiform larvae in direct wet mount preparation or by using concentration methods. **Figure 12** shows rhabditiform larvae of *S. stercoralis*.

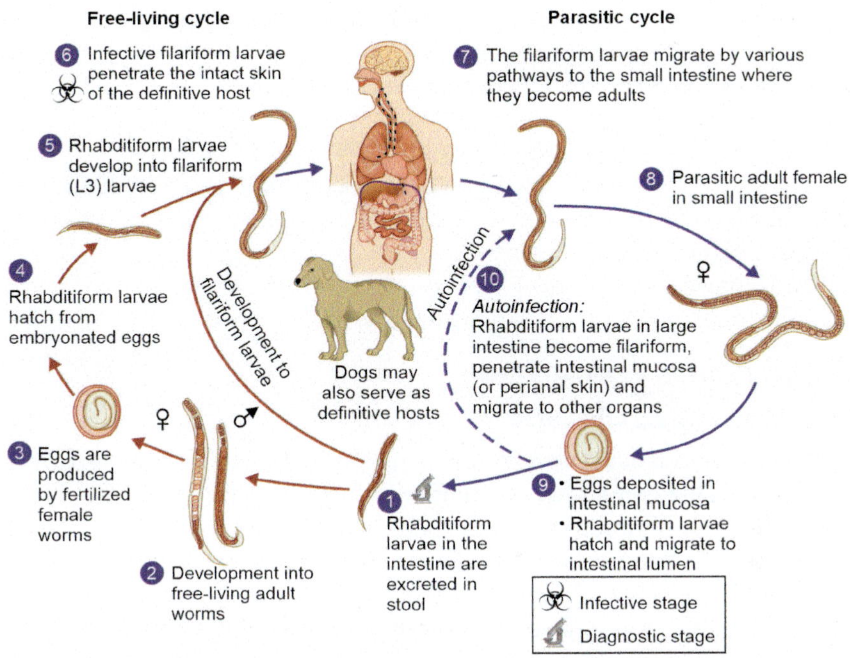

Fig. 11: Life cycle of *Strongyloides stercoralis*.
Source: Global Health, Division of Parasitic Diseases and Malaria https://www.cdc.gov/dpdx/strongyloidiasis/modules/Strongyloides_LifeCy also known as threadworm cle_lg.jpg

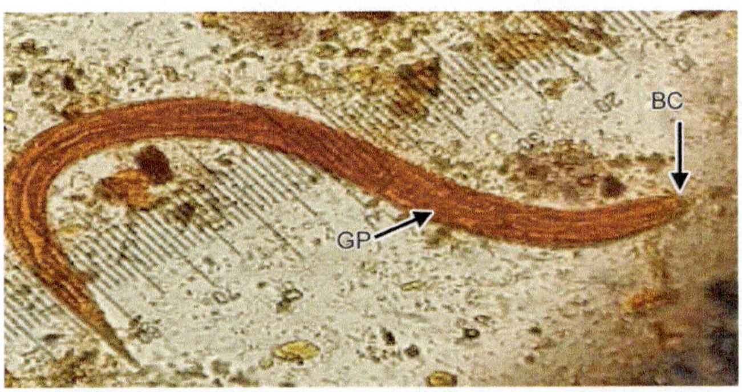

Fig. 12: *Strongyloides stercoralis rhabditiform* larvae (length 250 µm, magnification 40×). (BC: buccal cavity; GP: germinal primordium)
Source: Ottino L, Buonfrate D, Paradies P, Bisoffi Z, Antonelli A, Rossolini GM, et al. Pathogens | Free Full-Text | Autochthonous Human and Canine Strongyloides stercoralis Infection in Europe: Report of a Human Case in An Italian Teen and Systematic Review of the Literature (mdpi.com). Pathogens. 2020;9(6):439.

- Enterotest can be used.
- *Stool culture*: Agar plate culture and charcoal culture methods can be used.

- Serological tests such as ELISA and indirect hemagglutination using filarial antigens have been described.
- Complete blood count demonstrates eosinophilia (>500/cu.mm of blood)

Treatment

First line: Ivermectin 2 mg/kg PO for 2 consecutive days. Relatively contraindicated in pregnant or lactating women as safety profile not established (pregnancy category-C).
Albendazole 400 mg PO BD for 7 days. Its use is to be avoided in the first trimester of pregnancy (pregnancy category-C).[28]

ENTEROBIUS VERMICULARIS

Organism and its Life Cycle

Enterobius vermicularis also known as pinworm, threadworm or seatworm infection occurs commonly in children or institutionalized persons and is one of the most common worm infections in the United States.[29] Humans are considered the only hosts for pinworms. **Figures 13A and B** show the adult male worm and eggs under a microscope.

Humans become infected by ingesting embryonated eggs adhered to the nails while scratching perianal skin called self-inoculation or through exposure to contaminated bed linen and clothes. Once ingested, the eggshell gets dissolved in the stomach and larvae migrate to the cecum and appendix and mature into adult males measuring 2–5 mm and female worms measuring 8–13 mm within 15–30 days of infection. Adult male dies after copulation and female worms migrate to perianal skin at night, lay around 10,000 eggs, and subsequently die.[30] Eggs hatch into infective larvae within a few hours and may enter the intestine directly via the anus, a process called retroinfection. The eggs being resistant to desiccation will infect bedding and clothes. **Figure 14** depicts the life cycle of *Enterobius vermicularis.*

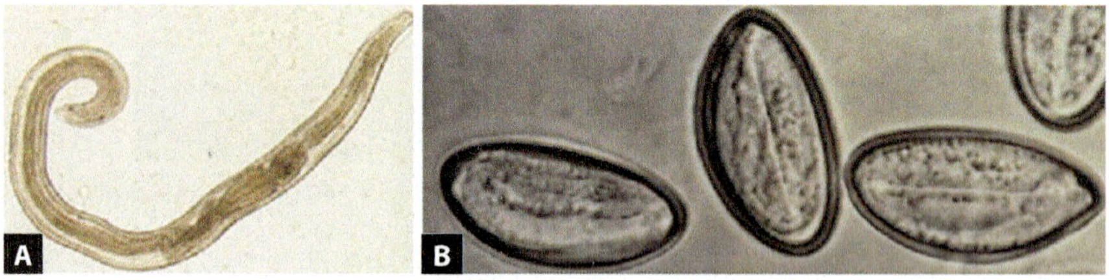

Figs. 13A and B: (A) Adult male of *Enterobius vermicularis* from a formalin-ethyl acetate (FEA) concentrated stool smear. The worm measured 1.4 mm in length. Image courtesy of Centre for Tropical Medicine and Imported Infectious Diseases; (B) Image of the eggs of the human parasite *E. vermicularis*, or "human pinworm," captured on cellulose tape under significant magnification. *Source:* DPDx, PHIL. Enterobiasis. [Online] Available from https://www.cdc.gov/parasites/pinworm/ [Last accessed November, 2024].

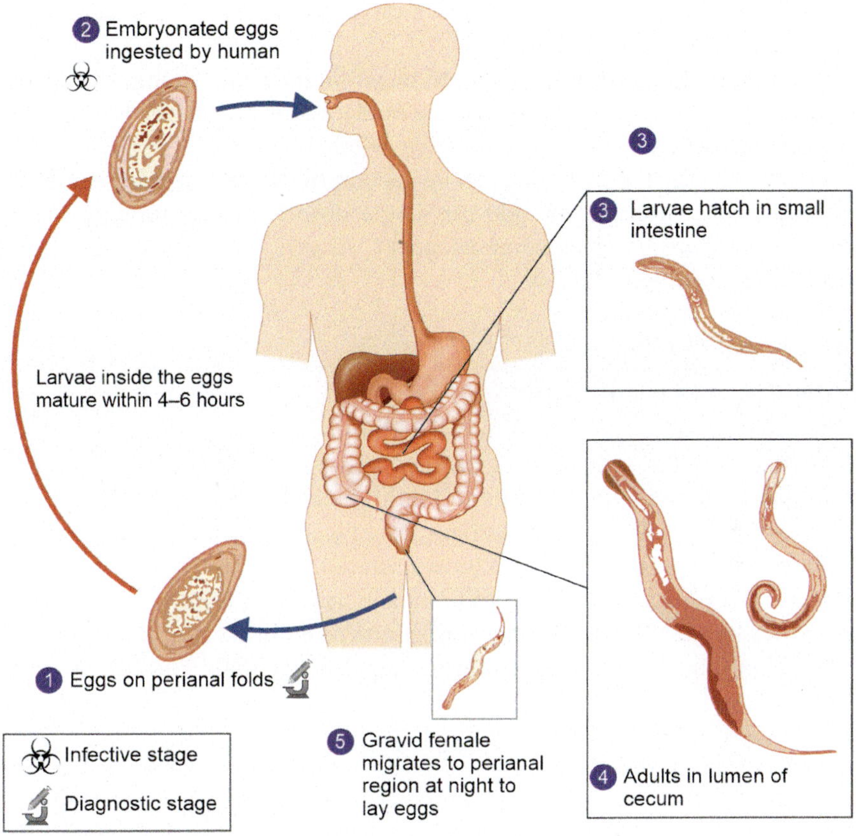

Fig. 14: Life cycle of *Enterobius vermicularis*.
Source: Global Health, Division of Parasitic Diseases and Malaria. About Pinworm Infection. [Online] Available from https://www.cdc.gov/parasites/pinworm/biology.html [Last accessed November, 2024].

Clinical Manifestations

Enterobiasis being usually asymptomatic rarely causes any complications in pregnant women. The most common symptom is nocturnal perineal itching and scratching of the anal area may lead to secondary bacterial infection. It may also present with abdominal pain, nausea, and anorexia in some cases. Complications such as appendicitis, endometritis, chronic salpingitis, vaginitis, urethritis, or intestinal ulceration may occur.[31]

Diagnosis and Treatment

Anal or perianal specimens are collected with the help of a cellophane swab, scotch tape, or NIH swab and observed for *Enterobius* eggs. Perianal samples are best collected in the morning and at least three scotch tapes are to be collected for 3 consecutive days which provides around 99% sensitivity.

Treatment for enterobiasis should be withheld until the third trimester or until delivery. Mebendazole 100 mg orally that is repeated 2 weeks later (pregnancy category-C).

Pyrantel pamoate 11 mg/kg can be used in the second or third trimester of pregnancy. Albendazole 400 mg single dose PO to be repeated after 2 weeks. They are also pregnancy category C drugs and should be used only if the benefit outweighs the risk.

TRICHURIS TRICHIURA

Organism and its Life Cycle

Trichuriasis being one of the most common soil-transmitted helminth infections is quite prevalent in tropical and subtropical areas with poor sanitation and hygiene as warm and humid climates are favorable for egg maturation. Infection occurs by ingestion of water and food contaminated with embryonated eggs. An egg is brown colored, bile staining, barrel-shaped with mucus plus at both ends and floats in saturated NaCl solution. After ingestion, larvae are released from the egg and pass down to the large intestine where they mature and develop into adult male and female worms. The adult worm measures around 40 mm in length and has a characteristic whip-like anterior shape, hence the name whipworm. The anterior thin part penetrates the mucosa and remains embedded there. Female worm after fertilization produces 5,000–7,000 eggs daily for up to 5 years. The eggs released fresh are unembryonated and noninfective and require incubation for around 3 weeks in the soil to become embryonated and infective. **Figure 15** shows the life cycle of *T. trichiura*.

Clinical Manifestations

Usually, light infections (100–200 worms) are asymptomatic and may cause nausea, headache, abdominal pain, and diarrhea in children with moderate infections (>200). Infections with above 800 worms may cause anemia or rectal prolapse or growth retardation. Iron deficiency anemia may develop due to heavy infection which is sufficient to cause bleeding in pregnant women.[32]

Diagnosis and Treatment

Stool Examination

- *Microscopy:* Characteristic barrel-shaped eggs identified on stool examination under a light microscope. **Figure 16** shows the egg of *T. trichiura* on an unstained wet mount.
- Blood examination shows eosinophilia

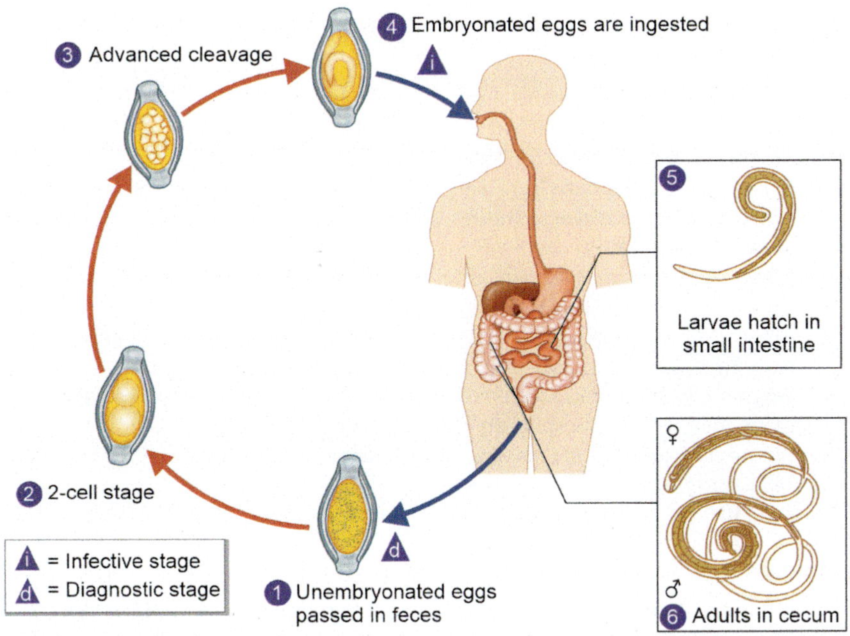

Fig. 15: Life cycle of *Trichuris trichiura*.
Source: Global Health, Division of Parasitic Diseases and Malaria. Trichuriasis. [Online] Available from https://www.cdc.gov/dpdx/trichuriasis/index.html?msclkid=d8fe1069a9d811ecb071fc1b739ba5af [Last accessed November, 2024].

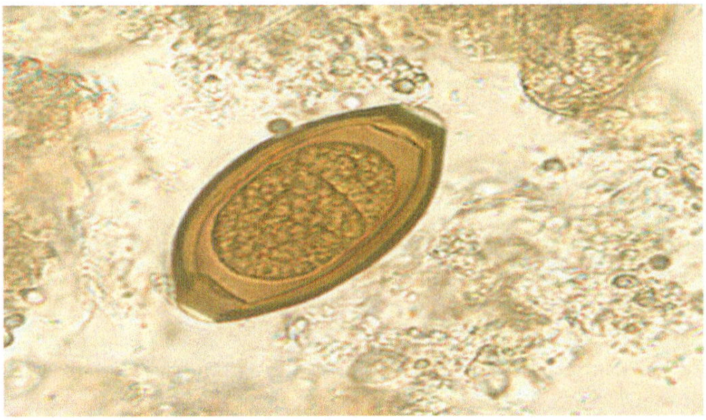

Fig. 16: Egg of *Trichuris trichiura* in an unstained wet mount.
Source: Global Health, Division of Parasitic Diseases and Malaria https://www.cdc.gov/dpdx/trichuriasis/images/1/Trichuris_trichiura_egg2.jpg

- Treatment in pregnancy should be deferred until after delivery. Mebendazole is the drug of choice given as 100 mg BD for 3 days. Alternatively, albendazole 400 mg daily for 3 days can be given.[33]

REFERENCES

Entamoeba histolytica

1. Elsdon-Dew R. The epidemiology of amoebiasis. Adv Parasitol. 1968:6:1-62.
2. Krogstad DJ, Spencer HC Jr, Healy GR. Current concepts in parasitology. Amebiasis. N Engl J Med. 1978;298(5):262-5.
3. Krogstad DJ, Spencer HC, Healy GR, Gleason NN, Sexton DJ, Herron CA. Amebiasis: epidemiologic studies in the United States, 1971-1974. Ann Intern Med. 1978;88(1):89-97.
4. Rivera R. Fatal postpartum amoebic colitis with trophozoites present in peritoneal fluid. Gastroenterology. 1972;62(2):314-7.
5. Abjoye AA. Fatal amoebic colitis in pregnancy and puerperium: a new clinico-pathological entity. J Trop Med Hyg. 1973;76(4):97-100.
6. Wagner VP, Smale LE, Lischke JH. Amebic abscess of the liver and spleen in pregnancy and the puerperium. Obstet Gynecol. 1975;45(5):562-5.
7. Charles D. Infections in Obstetrics and Gynecology. Philadelphia: WB Saunders; 1980. pp. 86-9.
8. Kean BH. The treatment of amebiasis. A recurrent agony. JAMA. 1976;235(5):501.

Giardia lamblia Infection

9. Brady PG, Wolfe JC. Waterborne giardiasis. Ann Intern Med. 1974;81(4):498-9.
10. Centers for Disease Control. Foodborne & Waterborne Disease Outbreaks Annual Summary 1976. Atlanta: Centers for Disease Control; 1977.
11. Wolfe MS. Giardiasis. N Engl J Med. 1978;298(6):319-21.
12. Walzer PD, Wolfe MS, Schultz MG. Giardiasis in travelers. J Infect Dis. 1971;124(2):235-7.
13. Black RE, Dykes AC, Sinclair SP, Wells JG. Giardiasis in day-care centers: Evidence of person-to-person transmission. Pediatrics. 1977;60(4):486-91.
14. Hoskins LC, Winawer SJ, Broitman SA, Gottlieb LS, Zamcheck N. Clinical giardiasis and intestinal malabsorption. Gastroenterology. 1967;53:265-79.

Infection with Intestinal Nematodes

15. Warren KS. Helminthic diseases endemic in the United States. Am J Trop Med Hyg. 1974;23:723-30.
16. Blumenthal DS. Intestinal nematodes in the United States. N Engl J Med. 1977;297(26):1437-9.
17. Spillman RK. Pulmonary ascariasis in tropical communities. Am J Trop Med Hyg. 1975;24(5):791-800.
18. Louw JH. Abdominal complications of Ascaris lumbricoides infestation in children. Br J Surg. 1966;53(6):510-21.
19. Blumenthal DS, Schultz MG. Incidence of intestinal obstruction in children infected with Ascaris lumbricoides. Am J Trop Med Hyg. 1975;24(5):801-5.
20. Tripathy K, Gonzales F, Lotero H, Bolaños O. Effects of Ascaris infection on human nutrition. Am J Trop Med Hyg. 1971;20(2):212-8.
21. Whittaker SG, Faustman EM. The effects of antitubuline agents on rat embryonic midbrain (CNS) cell cultures. Teratology. 1991;43:459.
22. Whittaker SG, Seely MR, Faustman EM. The effects of albendazole and albendazole sulfoxide on cultures of differentiating rat embyro limb bud cells. Teratology. 1990;41:598.

23. Banwell JG, Schad GA. Hookworm. Clin Gastroenterol. 1978;7(1):129-56.
24. Melvin DM, Brooke MM. Laboratory Procedures for the Diagnosis of Intestinal parasites, Publication no. CDC 75-8282. Washington, DC, US Department of Health, Education, and Welfare; 1974. p. 158.
25. Jones CA. Clinical studies in human strongyloidiasis, part I. Semeiology. Gastroenterology. 1950;16(4):743-56.
26. Milner PF, Irvine RA, Carton CJ et al: Intestinal malabsorption in Strongyloides stercoralis infestation. Gut. 1965;6(6):574-81.
27. Rivera E, Maldonado N, Velez-Garcia E, Grillo AJ, Malaret G. Hyperinfection syndrome with Strongyloides stercoralis. Ann Intern Med. 1972;72:199-204.
28. Purtilo DT, Meyers WM, Connor DH. Fatal strongyloidiasis in immunosuppressed patients. Am J Med. 1974;56(4):488-93.
29. Boyer A, Berdknikoff IK. Pinworm infestation in children: The problem and its management. Can Med Assoc J. 1962;86(2):60-5.
30. Simon RD. Pinworm infestation and urinary tract infection in young girls. Am J Dis Child. 1974;128(1):21-2.
31. Brooks TJ, Goetz CC, Plauche WC. Pelvic granuloma due to Enterobius vermicularis. JAMA. 1962;179:492-4.
32. Layrisse M, Aparcedol L, Martinez-Torres C, Roche M. Blood loss due to infection with Trichuris trichiura. Am J Trop Med Hyg. 1967;16(5):613-9.
33. Most H. Current concept in parasitology: Trichinosis—Preventable yet still with us. N Engl J Med. 1978;298:1178-80.

CHAPTER

6 *Trichomonas vaginalis* Infection

INTRODUCTION

Trichomoniasis is one of the most common sexually transmitted diseases caused by *Trichomonas vaginalis* which is a flagellated protozoan which resides in lumen of urogenital tract. Annually, an estimated 150 million people worldwide get infected.[1]

T. vaginalis is a pear-shaped flagellated protozoan which occurs only in a trophozoite stage with five flagella and characteristic twitching and erratic motility.[7] Females act as a reservoir of infection to man.[2] Parasite obtains nourishment from mucosal surface of vagina, remains adherent to it, cause superficial lesions and reproduce by longitudinal binary fission. Trophozoites are transmitted to male after sexual contact with infected female and localizes in urethra and prostate glands. **Figure 1** shows the lifecycle of *Trichomonas vaginalis*.

Growth of *T. vaginalis* is stunted a high oxygen pressure as it is a facultative anaerobe due to catalase deficiency. The trichomoniasis results in a higher pH around 5.5–7.0.[3]

EPIDEMIOLOGY

The incidence of trichomoniasis is 5–10% in healthy women while it may rise to 50–70% in female prison inmates and commercial sex workers. Risk factors for *T. vaginalis* infection include people with new or multiple sex partners, poor hygiene, low socioeconomic status, concurrent or history of other sexually transmitted diseases and unprotected sexual intercourse. The trichomonal infection usually peaks at the age of 16–35 years.

CLINICAL MANIFESTATIONS

Parasite mainly infects squamous epithelia of vagina in females.[3] Bartholin's gland, Skene's gland, and urethra may be infected. The most prevalent site of infection in men is the urethra[8] whereas prostatic secretions, epididymal aspirates, and seminal vesicles have also yielded *T. vaginalis*.[4]

Clinically, disease range from asymptomatic carrier state to severe vaginitis. This infection causes profuse vaginal discharge during pregnancy. Estrogens might promote parasite growth in vitro, which could justify the disease severity and persistence of infection in infected pregnant women or those using exogenous estrogens.[5,6]

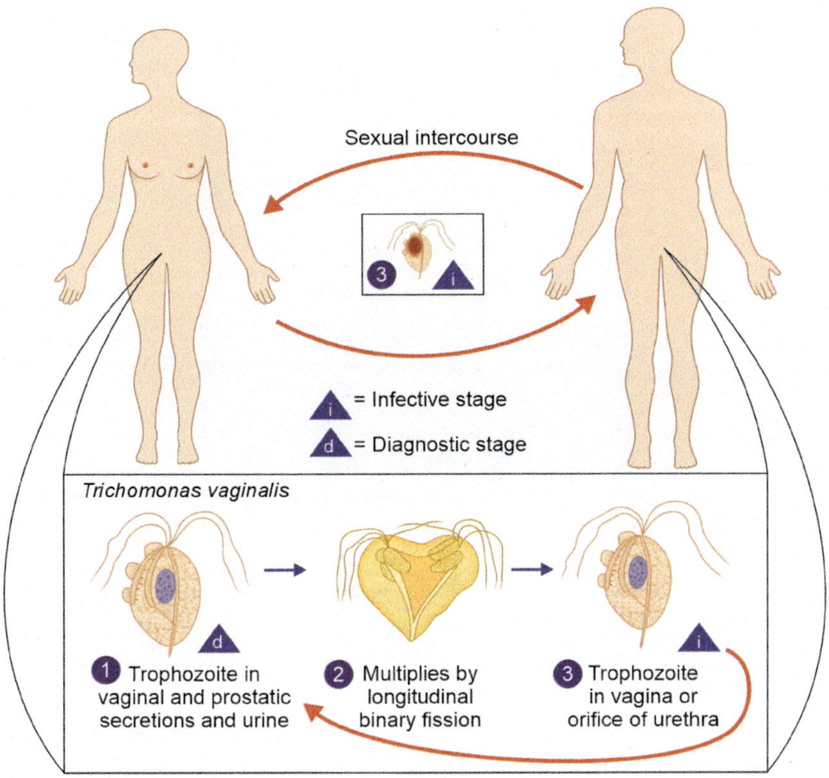

Fig. 1: Lifecycle of *Trichomonas vaginalis*.
Source: DPDx, CDC. Trichomoniasis. [online] Available from https://www.cdc.gov/dpdx/trichomoniasis/index.html?msclkid=d09d5d86a9fa11ecaa82f766b704f28d [Last accessed November, 2024]

In symptomatic women, malodorous purulent abnormal vaginal discharge, dyspareunia, and dysuria, lower abdominal pain, vulvovaginal irritation or itching. Postcoital bleeding may occur, which could be caused by *T. vaginalis* or other pathogens causing cervicitis.

Pelvic examination might reveal purulent vaginal discharge which can be characterized as a malodorous, thin, frothy yellow-green homogeneous discharge. Vulva, vagina, and cervix may be erythematous and edematous. Cervix may show small punctate hemorrhages called as "strawberry cervix" or "colpitis macularis" in around 40% of cases. **Figure 2** shows strawberry cervix appearance in *Trichomonas* infection.

INFECTION IN NEONATES

T. vaginalis infect around 2–17% of female neonates born to mother with vaginal infection.[9] In these infants, due to the influence of maternal estrogen, neonatal vaginal epithelium becomes relatively making them susceptible to trichomonial infection. By 3–4 weeks of age, maternal estrogen

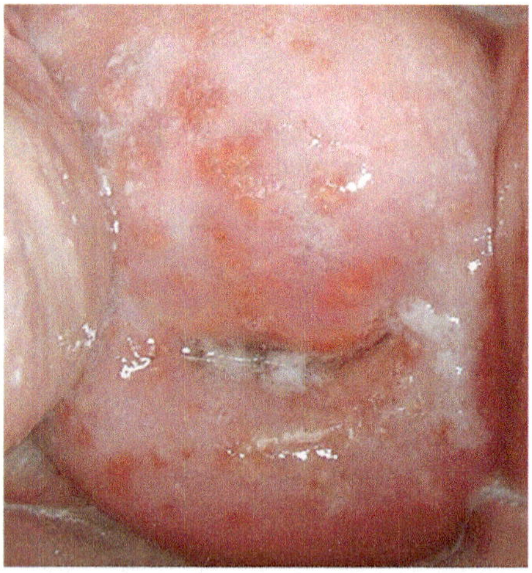

Fig. 2: Strawberry cervix in *Trichomonas vaginalis* infection, with inflammation and punctate hemorrhages (Reference from CMDT).

gets metabolized thus making vaginal epithelium in infants return to its comparatively resistant prepubescent state.

DIAGNOSIS

- *Sample:* Urogenital swabs of urinary sediments or vaginal secretion in females.
- *Microscopy:* On wet mount examination, pear-shaped flagellated trichomonads with characteristic jerky motility can be seen. Special stains like Papanicolaou, Giemsa can be used. Overall sensitivity of saline wet mount preparation is 40–60% while in symptomatic patients it is 80–90%. **Figure 3** shows pear-shaped structure of *Trichomonas* under microscopy.
- Nucleic acid amplification tests (NAATs) are more specific and sensitive for diagnosis of *T. vaginalis*.
- Cultures for *T. vaginalis* can be used in asymptomatic women with negative wet mount examination.
- Whiff test may be positive but this is not specific for trichomoniasis.

TREATMENT

Metronidazole 500 mg BD for 7 days. Clotrimazole intravaginally at a dose of 100 mg HS for 2 weeks can be a safer alternative to metronidazole. Some clinicians avoid metronidazole during 1st trimester. Partner treatment should also be done simultaneously as partner serves as a source of reinfection or alleged treatment failure. Patient to be advised to abstain from sexual activity until both the partner and patient are treated and all symptoms have resolved. Patient should also be advised to abstain from alcohol during the duration of treatment.

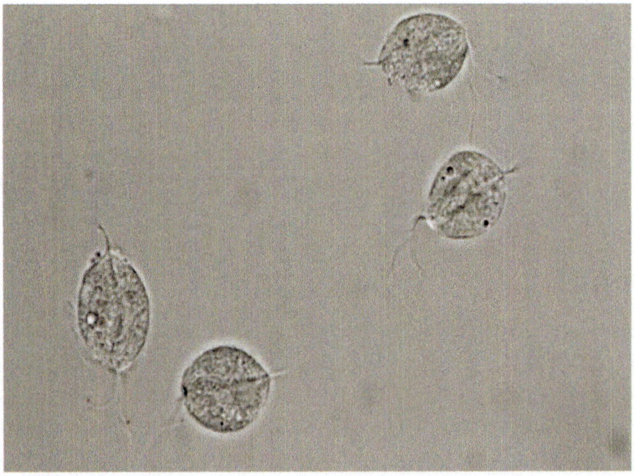

Fig. 3: Pear-shaped structures with small eccentrically placed nucleus as seen by wet mount microscopy.
Source: Šoba B, Skvarč M, Matičič M. Trichomoniasis: a brief review of diagnostic methods and our experience with real-time PCR for detecting infection. Acta Dermatovenerol Alp Pannonica Adriat. 2015;24(1):7-10.

Follow-up after 3 months and retesting after initial treatment as there are high chances of reinfection.

REFERENCES

1. Rowley J, Vander Hoorn S, Korenromp E, Low N, Unemo M, Abu-Raddad LJ, et al. Global and Regional Estimates of the Prevalence and Incidence of Four Curable Sexually Transmitted Infections in 2016. WHO Bulletin. [online] Available from https://www.who.int/bulletin/volumes/97/8/18-228486.pdf [Last accessed November, 2024].
2. Catterall RD. Trichomoniasis. Med Clin North Am. 1972;56:1203.
3. Rein MF, Chapel TA. Trichomoniasis, candidiasis, and the minor venereal diseases. Clin Obstet Gynecol. 1975;18:73.
4. Fouts AC, Kraus SJ. *Trichomonas vaginalis:* Re-evaluation of its clinical presentation and laboratory diagnosis. J Infect Dis. 1980;141:137.
5. Honigberg B, Brugerolle G. Trichomonads of importance in human medicine. In: Kreier JP (Ed). Parasitic Protozoa, Volume 2. New York: Academic Press; 1978. p. 275.
6. Al-Salihi FL, Curran JP, Wang J-S. Neonatal *Trichomonas vaginalis:* Report of 3 cases and review of the literature. Pediatrics. 1974;53:196.
7. Wisdon AR, Dunlop EMC. Trichomoniasis: Study of the disease and its treatment in women and men. Br J Vener Dis. 1965;41:990.
8. WHO. Non-gonococcal urethritis and other sexually transmitted diseases: Technical reprint series no. 816. Geneva: World Health Organization; 1981.
9. Rein MF, Muller M. *Trichomonas vaginalis*. In: Holmes KK, March PA, Sparling PF (Eds). Sexually transmitted diseases. New York: McGraw-Hill. 1990. pp. 481-92.

7 CHAPTER Trypanosomiasis

INTRODUCTION

Genus *Trypanosoma* consists of >20 species, of which only few are pathogenic to humans.[1] The trypanosomes which are pathogenic to humans are *Trypanosoma cruzi* causing Chagas disease (American trypanosomiasis) and two subspecies of *Trypanosoma brucei* namely *Trypanosoma brucei gambiense* causing chronic African trypanosomiasis (West African trypanosomiasis) and *Trypanosoma brucei rhodesiense* causing East African trypanosomiasis. Chagas disease is endemic in wildlife reservoirs throughout Americas, particularly rural impoverished areas in South and Central American countries. African trypanosomiasis is endemic in sub-Saharan African countries.[2]

ORGANISM AND ITS LIFE CYCLE

Trypanosomes have elongated, flattened leaf like, spindle-shaped body which is actively motile with the help of flagellum which originates from the kinetoplast at one end and connected along the length of body by an undulating membrane. Organism reproduces by binary longitudinal fission. **Figure 1** highlighting the structure of trypanosoma.

Life cycle varies in different species with man and domestic animals serving as primary host and blood sucking insects as the intermediate host.

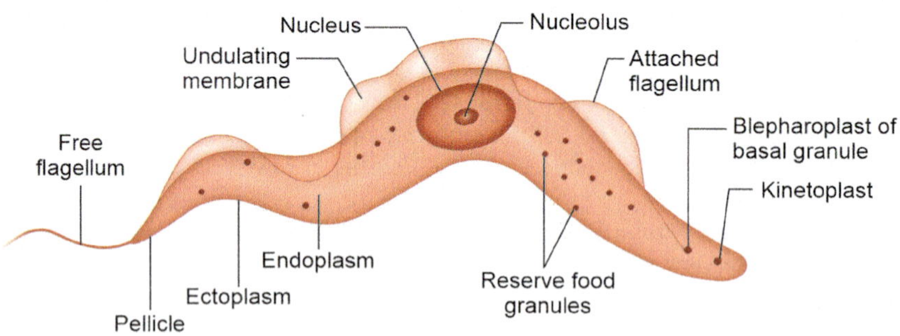

Fig. 1: Structure of a trypanosoma.
Source: Medhekar A. Structure and life cycle of trypanosome (with diagram). [online] Available from https://www.biologydiscussion.com/articles/structure-and-life-cycle-of-trypanosome-with-diagram/2681?msclkid=a79101ddaa9c11ec825261e3d9fcfe10 [Last accessed November, 2024].

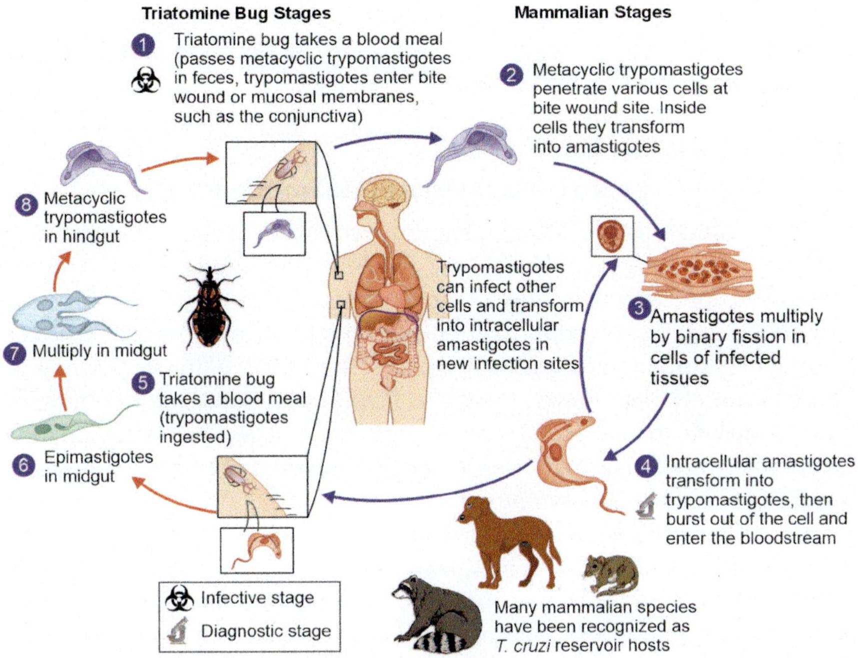

Fig. 2: Life cycle of *Trypanosoma cruzi*.
Source: DPDx. Global Health, division of parasitic diseases and malaria. [online] Available from https://www.cdc.gov/dpdx/trypanosomiasisamerican/index.html?msclkid=700b16a5aab311ec9cfdac7ac2590e8b [Last accessed November, 2024].

In African trypanosomiasis, *Glossina* species (tsetse fly) serves as a vector or intermediate host, while in Chagas' disease, reduviidae bugs (*Triatoma species*) serves the purpose. *T. cruzi* has cats, dogs, armadillos, woodrats, raccoons as reservoir host, *T. gambiense* has goats and cattle, while cattle and wild game animals are for *T. rhodesiense*. **Figure 2** shows life cycle of trypanosoma.

Infection begins by the bite of vector which causes injection of parasite or in the subcutaneous tissue where they actively multiply in tissue cells and intercellular spaces to form a chancre. Trypanosoma gain access to lymphatics and blood circulation and reproduce extensively by binary fission. While undergoing hematogenous dissemination, trypanosomes migrates to reticuloendothelial tissues or central nervous system (CNS), loses its flagella and undulating membrane and develop into leishmanial form. After some time, new flagellated forms are created, which can be consumed by the vector and start the process over again. Transplacental transmission is possible with all trypanosomes, resulting in in-utero fetal infection. Breast milk may contain infectious *T. cruzi*, which can spread to an infant via direct inoculation or the digestive tract. African trypanosomiasis during pregnancy can cause preterm labor, infertility, abortion, or stillbirth. Fertility and pregnancy are least affected in South American trypanosomiasis.

CLINICAL MANIFESTATIONS

West African Trypanosomiasis (*Trypanosoma gambiense*)

Incubation period is variable ranging from weeks to months. First sign after infection is a chancre of about 2–5 cm which develops at the site of bite and is erythematous and painful which becomes indurated and may ulcerate and blacken. Trypanosomes gain entry to lymphatics and multiply there leading to lymphadenitis appearing as a soft, mobile, painless swelling in the posterior cervical triangle known as "Winterbottom's sign." Intermittent fever, headache, malaise, myalgia, arthralgia, generalized lymphadenopathy, and hepatosplenomegaly are some of the features of first stage of disease. Neurologic or psychiatric symptoms and gastrointestinal symptoms may also be present. Kerandel's sign, which consists of severe pain after pressure of the palms or over the ulner nerve, may be present.

Second stage chronic phase of disease consist of CNS involvement-diffuse meningoencephalitis and meningomyelitis. Symptoms include headache, inability to concentrate, melancholic attitude, psychosis, tremors, ataxia, somnolence or insomnia, seizures ultimately leading to coma and death. Secondary infection such as malaria, dysentery, or aspiration pneumonia may occur which also increases mortality.

East African Trypanosomiasis (*T. rhodesiense*)

Incubation period ranges from a few days up to 3 weeks following which chancre may develop (more in travelers compared to natives). Disease has a fulminant course with severe febrile paroxysms, hemodynamic instability, thrombocytopenia, multiorgan failure, myocarditis, and disseminated intravascular coagulation.

Chagas' Disease (*T. cruzi*)

Disease occurs in acute and chronic phase. Acute phase which develops after an incubation period of 1–2 weeks, and lasting for 8–12 weeks is usually asymptomatic. However, there may be nonspecific symptoms such as abrupt onset fever, malaise, anorexia, erythematous rashes and cervical, axillary or iliac glands adenitis.

In some patients, there may be localized inflammation and induration at inoculation site of parasite known as Chagoma. Sometimes, parasite directly inoculates through mucosal surface like conjunctiva in case of which there occurs a characteristic edema of the orbital region referred to as *"Romaña's sign"* **(Fig. 3)**. Children mainly presents with acute form of disease.

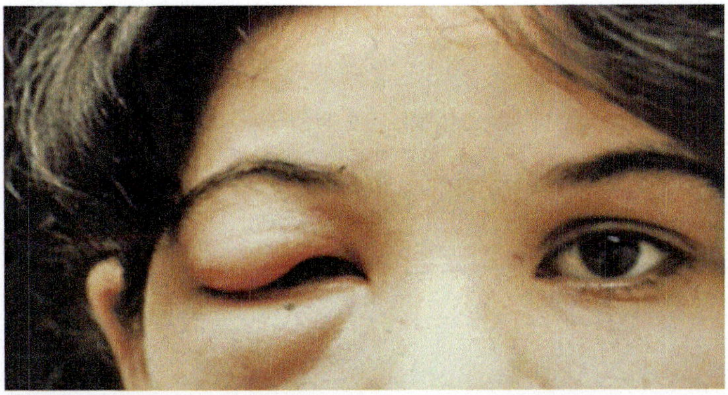

Fig. 3: Unilateral eyelid edema is the Romaña's sign of *Trypanosoma cruzi* infection. *Source:* Uptodate. Chagas disease. [online] Available from: https://www.uptodate.com/contents/image?imageKey=ID%2F58601&topicKey=ID%2F114181&search=chagas%20disease&rank=1~82&source=see_link [Last accessed November, 2024].

Severe disease is rare and may manifest as hepatosplenomegaly, myocarditis, congestive heart failure, pericardial effusion or meningoencephalitis.

In patients having indeterminate form of Chagas' disease, chronic Chagas' disease develops more slowly and insidiously. Cardiomyopathies can be found in 20–30% of chronic illness patients, and gastrointestinal symptoms, mostly related to the megaesophagus or megacolon, can be found in 10–15%.[1]

DIAGNOSIS

Microscopy

For diagnosis, organism is demonstrated in body fluids such as blood, cerebrospinal fluid (CSF), or in tissues with the help of microscope as seen in **Figure 4**. Blood examination include direct thin peripheral smear or Giemsa stained thick or thin smear. Specimen may be concentrated for better yield in case of Gambiense trypanosomiasis with the help of buffy coat separation, anion exchange centrifugation and hematocrit centrifugation methods.[3]

Tissue aspirate from enlarged cervical lymph node may demonstrate motile trypanosomes on direct wet mount with ground glass illumination.

For chronic disease, serology is preferred as trypanosomes are rarely present in blood circulation due to low parasitemia. Enzyme immune assay (EIA) based on recombinant *T. cruzi* antigen and immunoblot assay using trypomastigote excreted-secreted antigens (TESA-blot) are used as first line tests. Immunofluorescence assay and enzyme-linked immunosorbent assay (ELISA) can also be used. **Figure 5** showing immunofluorescent assay.

Rapid diagnostic tests: Card agglutination test for trypanosomiasis (CATT)

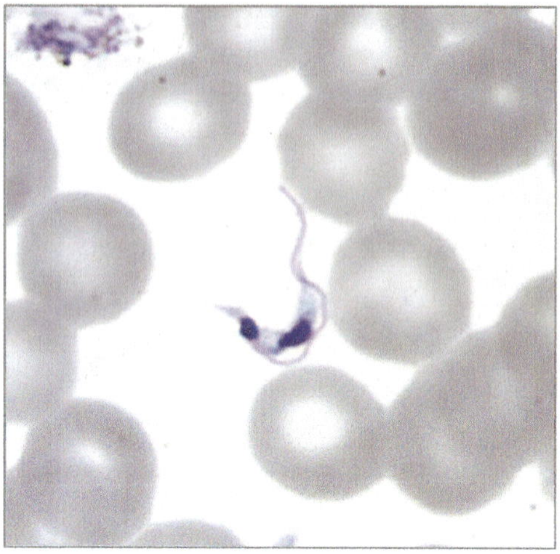

Fig. 4: *T. cruzi* trypomastigote in a thin blood smear stained with Giemsa. Note the typical C-shape of the trypomastigote that characterizes *T. cruzi* in fixed blood smears. *Source:* DPDx. Global Health, Division of Parasitic Diseases and Malaria. [online] Available from: https://www.cdc.gov/dpdx/trypanosomiasisamerican/images/2/Tcruzi_thin_giemsa_subt.jpg https://www.cdc.gov/dpdx/trypanosomiasisamerican/index.html?msclkid=700b16a5aab311ec9cfdac7ac2590e8b [Last accessed November, 2024].

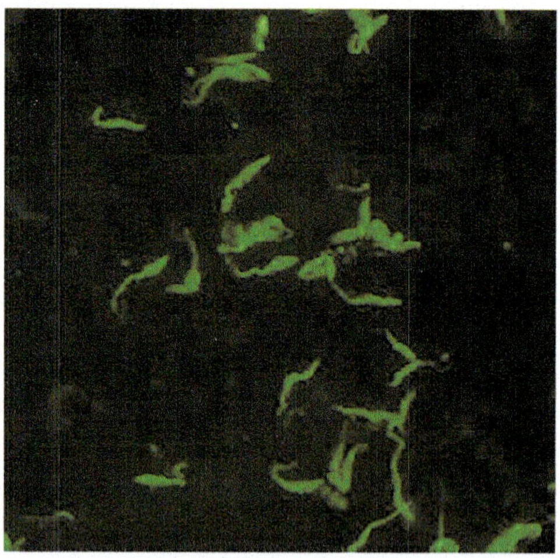

Fig. 5: Positive IFA result with *T. cruzi* antigen (magnification 400x)
Source: DPDx. Global Health, Division of Parasitic Diseases and Malaria. [online] Available from https://www.cdc.gov/dpdx/trypanosomiasisamerican/index.html?msclkid=700b16a5aab311ec9cfdac7ac2590e8b [Last accessed November, 2024].

TREATMENT

For *T. Gambiense* infection in first stage, pentamidine is used. Suramin can also be used but is generally avoided in *Gambiense* infection due to risk of severe adverse reactions in patients coinfected with onchocerciasis which usually occurs in *T. gambiense* endemic areas. Second stage gambiense is treated with nifurtimox-eflornithine combination therapy (NECT). Fexinidazole is newer drug for gambiense infection approved for use in rural areas of Africa.

For *T. rhodesiense*, suramin is the first line drug for first stage disease which can be given after a 100–200-mg test dose in a dose of 1g given intravenously on the 1st, 3rd, 7th, 14th, and 21st days, for a total of 5 g. For second stage disease when CNS involvement occurs, melarsoprol (Mel B) is used along with steroids to prevent encephalopathy caused by melarsoprol.

Nifurtimox and benznidazole can be used for treatment. These drugs are contraindicated in severe hepatic or renal disease. Nifurtimox is given at a dose of 8–10 mg/kg/day PO in three divided doses for 2 months. Benznidazole can be used at a dose of 5–8 mg/kg/day PO in two divided doses for 2 months. Both the drugs are pregnancy category-NA may be possibly toxic to pregnancy, however, as infection is severe and life threatening, their use is warranted in pregnancy.

REFERENCES

1. Rassi A Jr, Rassi A, Marin-Neto JA. Chagas disease. Lancet. 2010;375(9723):1388.
2. DeRaadt P. African sleeping sickness today. Trans R Soc Trop Med Hyg. 1976;70(2):114.
3. Eyckman L. *Trypanosoma* species. In: Mandel GL, Douglas RG, Bennett JE (Eds). Principles and practice of infectious diseases. New York: John Wiley & Sons; 1980. pp. 2118-27.

8

CHAPTER

Leishmaniasis

ORGANISM AND ITS LIFE CYCLE (FIG. 1)

Leishmaniasis is a complex of several vector borne disease caused by an obligate intracellular protozoa of genus *Leishmania*. Symptoms range from cutaneous ulcers to multisystem disease. It is spread with the bite of an infected female sandfly *Phlebotomus* to mammalian hosts such as rodents, wild or domestic canines, and humans being the accidental host due to

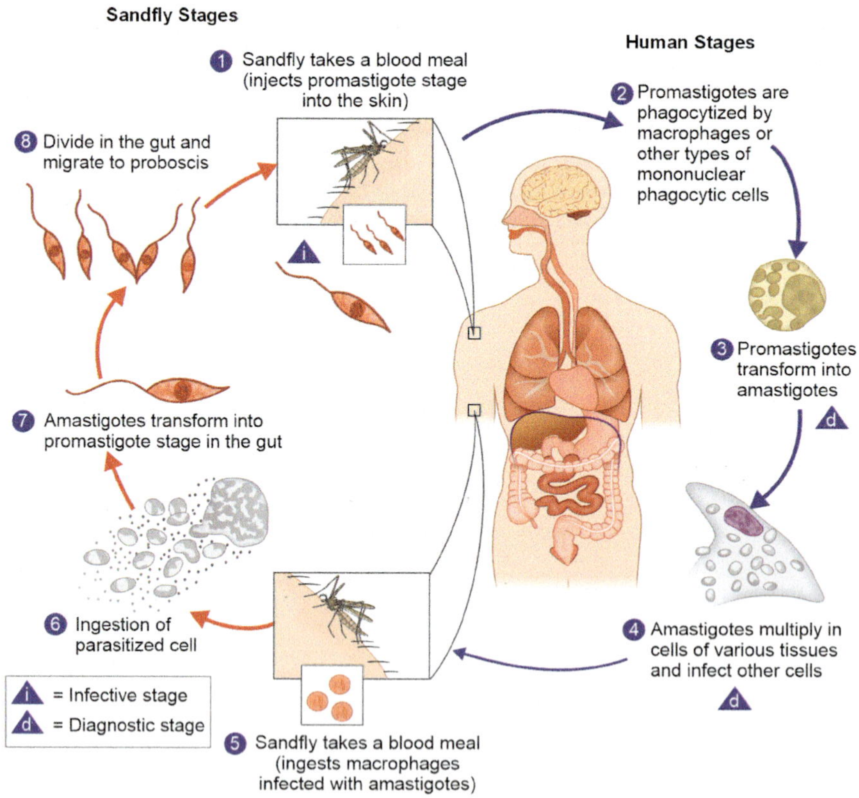

Fig. 1: Life cycle of *Leishmania*.
Source: DPDx. Global Health, Division of Parasitic Diseases and Malaria. [online] Available from https://www.cdc.gov/dpdx/leishmaniasis/ [Last accessed November, 2024].

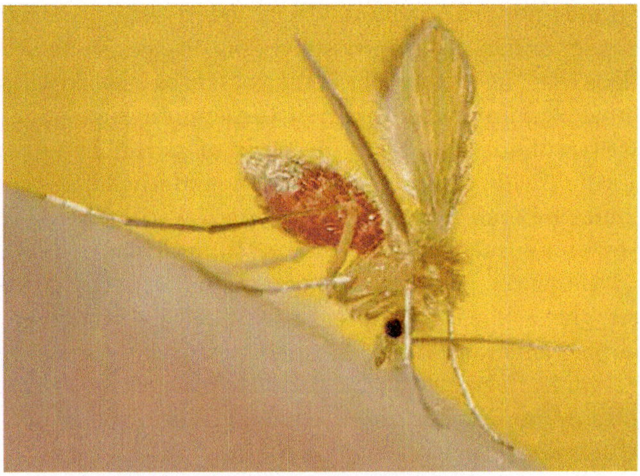

Fig. 2: Sandfly *Phlebotomus* species.
Source: DPDx. Global Health, Division of Parasitic Diseases and Malaria.

presence in endemic areas. Its treatment is expensive and control of disease can be aimed by eliminating its vector.[1] It is widespread in Europe, Africa, India, Afghanistan, Pakistan, Syria, and the Western Hemisphere, as well as regions of Central and South America, and produces the disease kala-azar. *Leishmania tropica*, *Leishmania major* are the classical form or old world leishmaniasis (Oriental sore) while *Leishmania braziliensis* and *Leishmania mexicana* (New World leishmaniasis) causes cutaneous or mucosal leishmaniasis with extensive destruction of nasal mucosa as well. Annual incidence of cutaneous leishmaniasis is 0.7–1 million cases.

Humans acquire the infection from the bite of infected female sandfly *Phlebotomus* **(Fig. 2)** and promastigote forms of parasite gain access to macrophages of reticuloendothelial system (*Leishmania donovani*) or histiocytes present in the dermis (cutaneous leishmaniasis). Promastigote form convert into amastigote forms in reticuloendothelial cells and divide by binary fission giving rise to daughter amastigotes which re invade neighboring histiocytes or in visceral leishmaniasis disseminate throughout reticuloendothelial system. Parasite present in infected skin or in blood is sucked up by the sandflies while biting humans for their blood meal. Inside the sandfly, parasites develop into infective promastigote form and again may transmit the infection to humans. **Figure 1** shows the life cycle of *Leishmania*.

CLINICAL MANIFESTATIONS

Visceral Leishmaniasis

Incubation period is of this disease ranges from 2 to 6 months but may vary from few weeks to years. Symptoms such as fever, malaise, abdominal pain, and fullness in left upper quadrant, weight loss usually occur and may be gradual in onset or may progress rapidly. This disease is characteristically known as "kala azar" referring to blackening of skin associated with infection.

Abdominal examination shows hepatosplenomegaly with abdominal tenderness, lymphadenopathy, with signs of portal hypotension and edema. Parasite divide extensively in reticuloendothelial system, leading to a high parasitic load in spleen, bone marrow and liver. Anemia and thrombocytopenia ensues with bone marrow suppression, hemolysis leading to hepatic dysfunction, jaundice, ascites, and hemorrhagic complications. The skin gets gray as the disease progresses, and light-skinned people may notice hyperpigmentation.[2] Most visceral leishmaniasis patients are cachexic and infertile, while pregnancy during the early stages of the disease involves a risk of intrauterine fetal infection.[3] Increased risk of abortion noted in infection with *L. donovoni.*

CUTANEOUS LEISHMANIASIS

L. tropica, L. braziliensis, and *L. mexicana* all display comparable clinical symptoms of cutaneous leishmaniasis. Disease begins as an erythematous papule at the site of bite which grows and form a nodule which further progresses to a painless ulceration with an indurated margin. The ulcerated area may become covered with hyperkeratotic hyperpigmented eschar. In *L. mexicana* and *L. braziliensis* infection, mucosal leishmaniasis consisting of mucosal destruction with symptoms such as nasal stuffiness, blockage, bleeding, increased secretions, sloughing of dead tissue and erosions in nose, mouth or nasal septum may occur up to 10 years or more following cutaneous leishmaniasis.

DIAGNOSIS

Microscopy

Amastigote forms are seen on examination of tissue specimens such as blood, bone marrow, lymph nodes, and splenic tissue with the help of Giemsa and H and E stain. **Figure 3** shows amastigote forms with Giemsa staining.

Serologic tests are not much helpful as most patient do not mount significant antibody response.

Culture is done on Novy-MacNeal-Nicolle (NNN) media which is a biphasic media.

Molecular diagnostic techniques like polymerase chain reaction (PCR) based technology is applied which has more sensitivity and is rapid.[4]

TREATMENT

Treatment should be postponed until after the baby is born. Patients with visceral leishmaniasis, on the other hand, must be treated right away, regardless of whether or not they are pregnant. For all kinds of leishmaniasis,

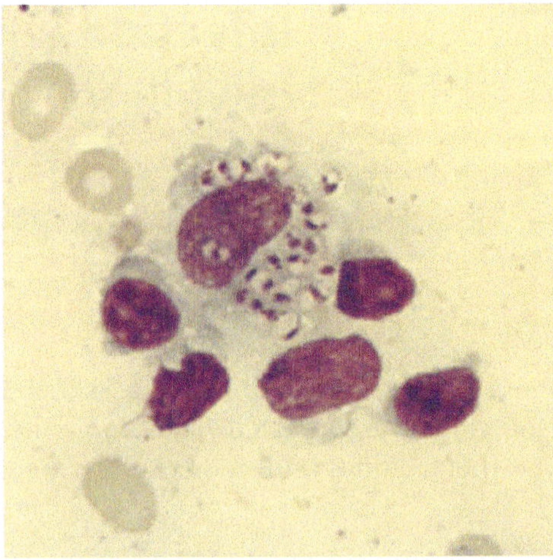

Fig. 3: *Leishmania* spp. amastigotes in a Giemsa-stained tissue scraping.
Source: DPDx. Global Health, Division of Parasitic Diseases and Malaria. [online] Available from: https://www.cdc.gov/dpdx/leishmaniasis/ [Last accessed November, 2024].

sodium stibogluconate (Pentostam) is the medication of choice. The adult dose for visceral leishmaniasis is 20 mg/kg/day, given in three doses intravenously or intramuscularly over the course of 20 days. The dose for cutaneous leishmaniasis is 0.6 g intramuscularly given for 10 days. Amphotericin B, 0.25–1 mg/kg intravenously daily or every other day for up to 8 weeks, should be given to patients who do not react to antimonials. Antimonials' toxicity during pregnancy is unknown.

REFERENCES

1. Laison R, Shaw JJ. Epidemiology and ecology of leishmaniasis in Latin America. Nature. 1978;273(5664):595-600.
2. Figueiró-Filho EA, Duarte G, El-Beitune P, Quintana SM, Maia TL. Visceral leishmaniasis (kala-azar) and pregnancy. Infect Dis Obstet Gynecol. 2004;12(1):31-40.
3. Low GC, Cook WE. A congenital case of kala-azar. Lancet. 1926;211:1209.
4. Deborggraeve S, Laurent T, Espinosa D, Van der Auwera G, Mbuchi M, Wasunna M, et al. A simplified and standardized polymerase chain reaction format for the diagnosis of leishmaniasis. J Infect Dis. 2008;198:1565-72.

9 CHAPTER

Infection with Tissue-dwelling Nematodes

INTRODUCTION

Tissue-dwelling nematodes are highly prevalent, especially in the tropics, where millions of individuals are infected. These organisms usually have a complicated life cycle that includes arthropods as intermediate hosts (except in *Trichinella*).

TRICHINOSIS

Humans acquire infection after ingesting raw or uncooked meat harboring live larvae. Once cyst wall gets digested in the stomach, larvae get releases and adhere to jejunal mucosa and mature into adult worms.[1] Female adult worm after fertilization releases around 500 larvae which causes parasitemia or larvae burrow into the muscle fiber where it gets encysted and become infective if ingested by another host. Bear, pigs, rats, and other wild animals act as a reservoir hosts for *Trichinella spiralis*. **Figure 1** depicts the life cycle of *Trichinella*. **Figure 2** shows bear muscle-encysted *Trichinella* larvae.

Clinical Manifestations

After ingestion of contaminated food, patients may develop nausea, vomiting, diarrhea, abdominal pain within 1–2 days. Within 2 weeks, patient may show symptoms such as fever, myalgia, orbital swelling, subconjunctival hemorrhage, chemosis, malaise, headache, macular or petechial rashes, diarrhea, or constipation. Some patients with heavy infection may show symptoms like cough, dyspnea, and sometimes death. Symptoms of mild-to-moderate infection may go away within a few months.[1]

Diagnosis and Treatment

Diagnosis is made based on history of consumption of meat with signs and symptoms suggestive of trichinosis. Eosinophilia may be seen on complete blood count examination.

Lab diagnosis is made by serological test like *Trichinella* antibody test (EIA) or by visualization of encysted larvae in a muscle biopsy sample.[2]

Treatment consists of albendazole at a dose of 400 mg BD for 8–14 days. Alternatively, mebendazole 200–400 mg PO TDS for 3 days followed by 400–500 mg PO TDS for 10 days. Steroids may be needed in severe cases.

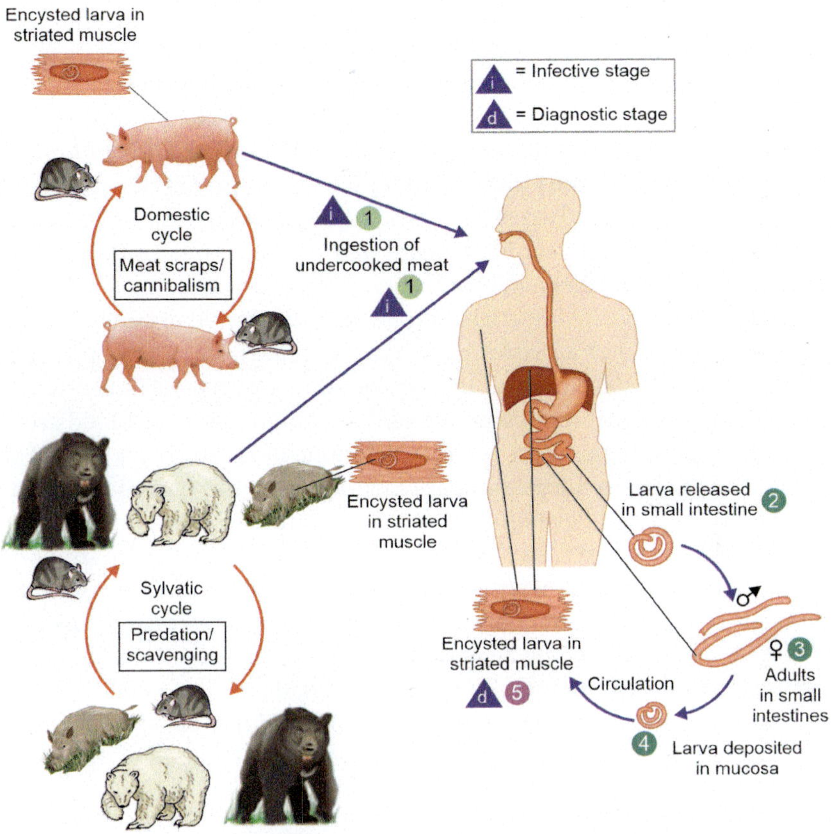

Fig. 1: Life cycle of *Trichinella spiralis*.
Source: CDC. Trichinella life cycle. [online] Available from: https://www.cdc.gov/parasites/images/trichinellosis/Trichinella_LifeCycle.gif [Last accessed November, 2024].

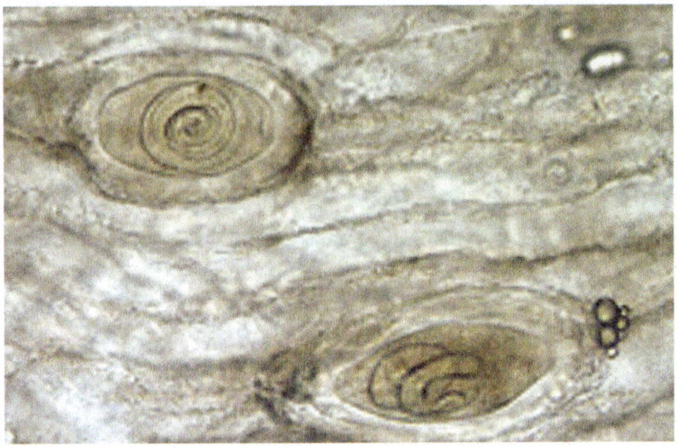

Fig. 2: Bear muscle showing encysted *Trichinella* larvae.
Source: CDC. Trichinellosis. [online] Available from: https://www.cdc.gov/parasites/trichinellosis/diagnosis.html [Last accessed November, 2024].

Both are pregnancy category C drugs. Can be given in second or third trimester of pregnancy after weighing the benefit-risk in pregnant females.

FILARIASIS

The filarial nematodes *Wuchereria bancrofti* and *Brugia malayi* are transmitted by mosquitos and cause Bancroftian and Malayan filariasis, respectively. There are two other filarial illnesses that are transmitted to humans by arthropod vectors: *Onchocerca volvulus* and *Loa loa*. These diseases do not affect pregnancy or the newborn in any way.[3]

Humans acquire the infection with the bite of infected arthropod vector, which transmits the infective form of larvae to skin. These larvae gain access to lymphatic and develop into threadlike adult worms. Fertilized female releases microfilariae into lymphatic and they then enter the bloodstream reaching the peripheral blood. Nocturnal periodicity is shown by *W. bancrofti* and *B. malayi*. These microfilaria are ingested by arthropod vector during their blood meal and develop further into the arthropod to infective larval stage which may again cause infection to host. Microfilariae are shed into the blood by *L. loa* adult worms while they are actively migrating through connective tissue. Adults frequently dwell in fibrous nodules (onchocercomas) in subcutaneous tissue and release unsheathed microflaria in blood that migrate to connective tissues. These microfilariae are consumed by female black flies and the cycle continues. **Figures 3A and B** show the life cycle of *B. malayi* and *W. bancrofti* species.

Clinical Manifestations

Even though microfilariae are present in bloodstream, infection by *W. bancrofti* and *B. malayi* are often asymptomatic. Acute inflammation or chronic lymphatic blockage are the most common causes of development of symptoms in this infection. Headache, nausea, fever, and backache and are common symptoms of lymphangitis or lymphadenitis and may cause secondary bacterial infection. In chronic cases, due to swelling and decreased lymphatic drainage owing to lymphatic drainage dysfunction, patients develop lymphedema mainly affecting the legs causing elephantiasis but can also develop in arms, breasts, and genitals leading to fertility and lactation issues. Vulval elephantiasis can lead to obstruction of labor and thus increasing chances of caesarean section. Filarial infection can also lead to tropical pulmonary eosinophilia which causes symptoms such as cough, dyspnea, wheezing, or hemoptysis with elevated eosinophil counts found on peripheral smear examination.[4]

L. loa infection usually presents with transient localized swelling around wrists and knees called "*Calabar swellings.*" A *loa loa* worm can be sometimes seen travelling through the eye's subconjunctiva. Onchocerciasis also called "river blindness" presents with nontender, mobile subcutaneous

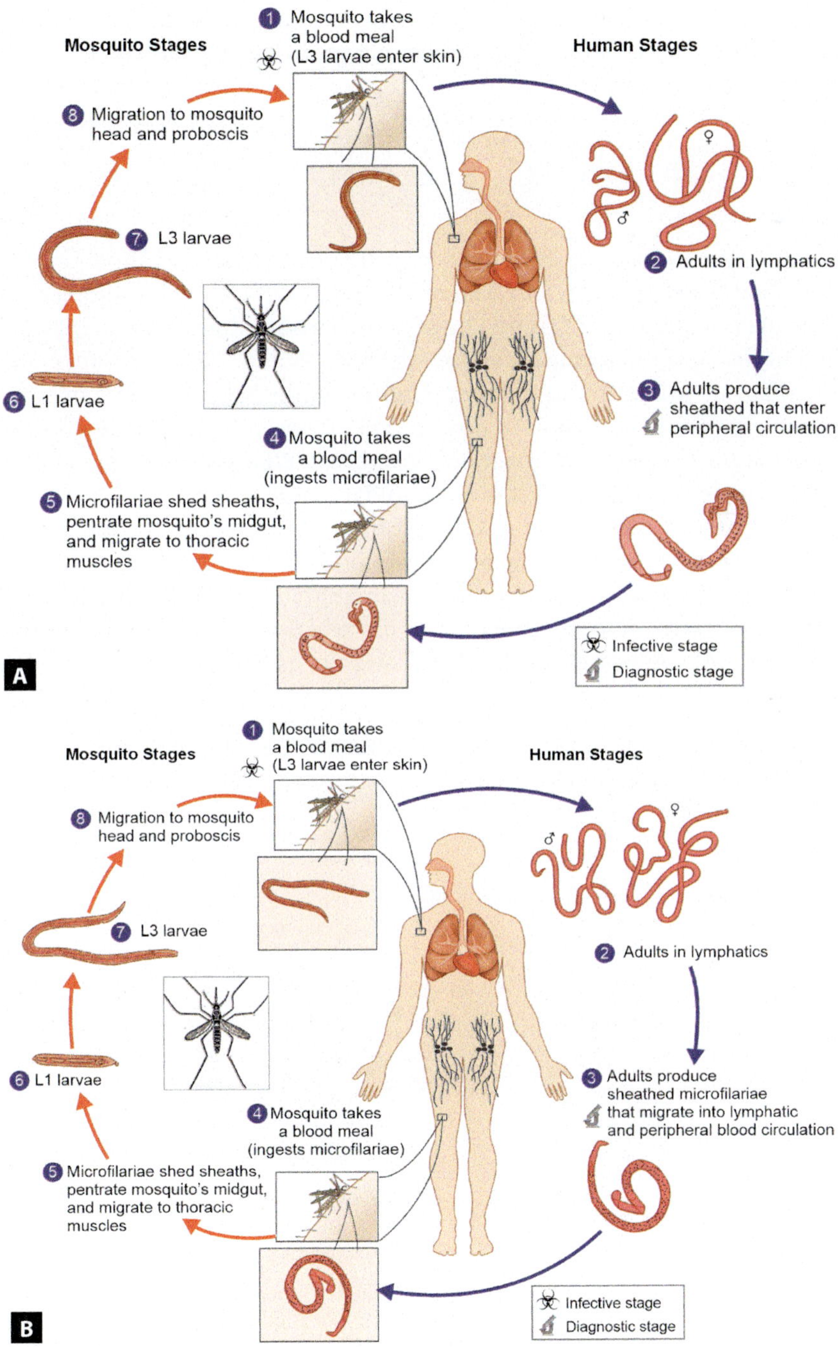

Figs. 3A and B: Life cycle of (A) *Brugia malayi* and (B) *Wuchereria bancrofti* species. *Source:* CDC. Lymphatic filariasis. [online] Available from: https://www.cdc.gov/parasites/lymphaticfilariasis/biology.html [Last accessed November, 2024].

nodules harboring worms, skin rashes along with itching leading to "leopard skin appearance" in some.[5] Onchocerca microfilariae may die in eye leading to clouding of cornea which may further progress to blindness, iridocyclitis, glaucoma, choroiditis, and optic atrophy.

Diagnosis and Treatment

Microscopy

Visualization of parasite in blood smear by microscopic examination. For identification of Malayan and bancroftian microfilariae, blood samples are best taken at midnight (10 PM–2 AM), concentrated using concentration techniques and thick smears are made, and stained. For *L. loa* infection, microfilariae are found in daytime blood sample. Microfilariae observed in skin snips or in cornea or in posterior chamber of the eye on a slit lamp examination are used to diagnose onchocerciasis. **Figure 4** shows microfilaria of *W. bancrofti* and **Figure 5** shows microfilaria of *B. malayi.*

Treatment should be delayed until after delivery unless symptoms are severe enough to require immediate treatment.

Treatment consists of diethylcarbamazine citrate except in onchocerciasis where it is contraindicated due to Mazzotti reaction-severe exacerbation of skin and eye involvement. It is microfilaricidal as well as effective against adult worm.

Dose: 6 mg/kg/day either on a single day or a 12 days treatment may be initiated. Therapy should be used for longer duration like 14–21 days in cases of tropical pulmonary eosinophilia.

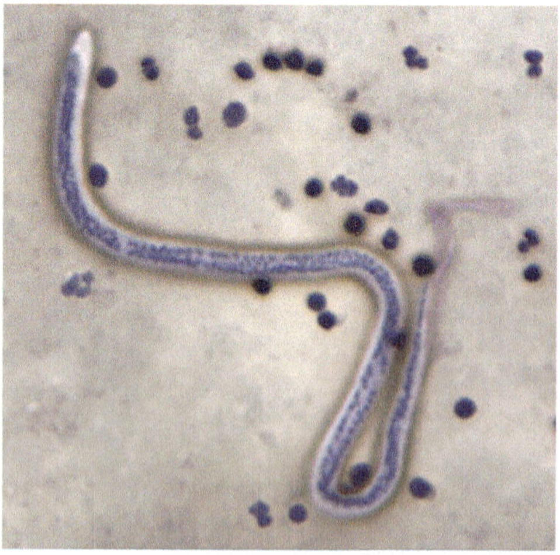

Fig. 4: Microfilaria of *Wuchereria bancrofti* in a thick blood smear stained with Giemsa.
Courtesy: Oregon State Public Health Laboratory.
Source: CDC. *Wuchereria bancrofti.* [online] Available from: https://www.cdc.gov/dpdx/lymphaticfilariasis/images/1/W_bancrofti_ORa.jpg [Last accessed November, 2024].

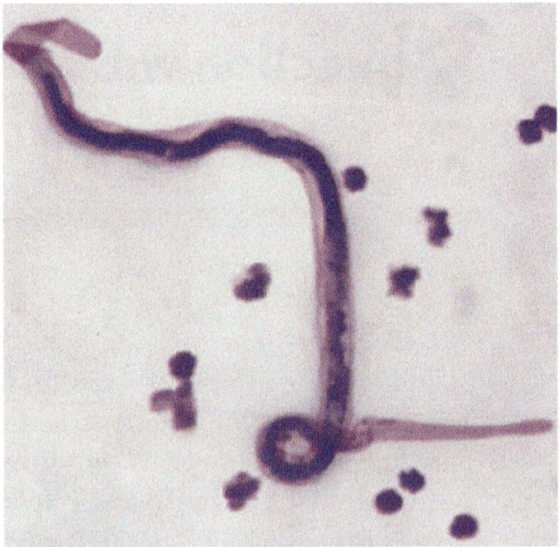

Fig. 5: Microfilaria of *B. malayi* in a thick blood smear, stained with Giemsa.
Source: CDC. Brugia Malayi. [online] Available from https://www.cdc.gov/dpdx/lymphaticfilariasis/images/3/Brugia_malayi.jpg [Last accessed November, 2024].

Alternatively, ivermectin can be used which is effective against microfilaria but not against adult worm. Ivermectin 150 g/kg orally once every 6–12 months is the standard treatment for onchocerciasis. Doxycycline 200 mg/day for 4–6 weeks kills adult worms too.

REFERENCES

1. Most H. Current concept in parasitology: Trichinosis. Preventable yet still with us. N Engl J Med. 1978;298(21):1178-80.
2. Gould SE. Trichinosis in Man and Animals. In: Gould SE (Ed). Springfield, IL: Charles C Thomas; 1970.
3. Neva FA, Ottesen EA. Current concepts in parasitology: Tropical (filarial) eosinophilia. N Engl J Med. 1978;298(20):1129-30.
4. Anderson J, Fuglsang H. Ocular onchocerciasis. Trop Dis Bull. 1972;74(4):257-72.

CHAPTER

10 Infection with Trematodes

INTRODUCTION

Trematodes are parasitic flukes with complex life cycles involving aquatic freshwater snails as intermediate hosts and humans and cattle, dogs, cats, and rodents serve as reservoir host. Adult worms reproduce sexually, while larvae reproduce asexually. Almost all the flukes infecting humans are hermaphrodites except *Schistosomes* which are dioecious containing both male and female worms. *Schistosoma, Clonorchis, Fasciolopsis, Opisthorchis, Fasciola,* and *Paragonimus* are some of the flukes causing disease in man.

SCHISTOSOMIASIS/BILHARZIASIS

Schistosomiasis infect about 200 million people globally with highest prevalence in sub-Saharan Africa, more in rural areas. Other places where schistosomiasis is common are South America, Middle East, Caribbean, Indonesia, and East Asia.[1] Three major species of *Schistosoma* affecting humans are *Schistosoma haematobium, Schistosoma mansoni,* and *Schistosoma japonicum. S. haematobium* affects people in sub-Saharan Africa, Middle East, Arabia while *S. mansoni* occurs in sub-Saharan Africa, Arabia, South America especially Brazil and Caribbean. Infection by *S. japonicum* is more prevalent in China, Philippines, and Indonesia.

Adult worms are cylindrical, bilaterally symmetrical and flattened dorsoventrally. Adult males have a groove like structure throughout the length which is called gynaecophoric canal in which female worm resides.

Infection is acquired by humans when *Cercariae* penetrate the skin from contaminated fresh water source and develop into schistosomule and migrate to liver through bloodstream. In liver, schistosomule develop into adult worms and travel against the bloodstream in the portal venous system to reach mesenteric veins of intestine (*S. mansoni* and *S. japonicum*) or vesical plexus (*S. haematobium*). The adult worms are dioecious and have a life span of 30 years. Female worms after fertilization deposits egg in mesenteric venules or perivesical veins. In *S. haematobium*, eggs are excreted through urine while in infections of *S. mansoni* and *S. japonicum*, it is passed through feces. These eggs after hatching in water releases miracidia which is motile and can live up to 7 days in water and infect snails. These miracidia undergo asexual multiplication in snails and releases *Cercariae* into

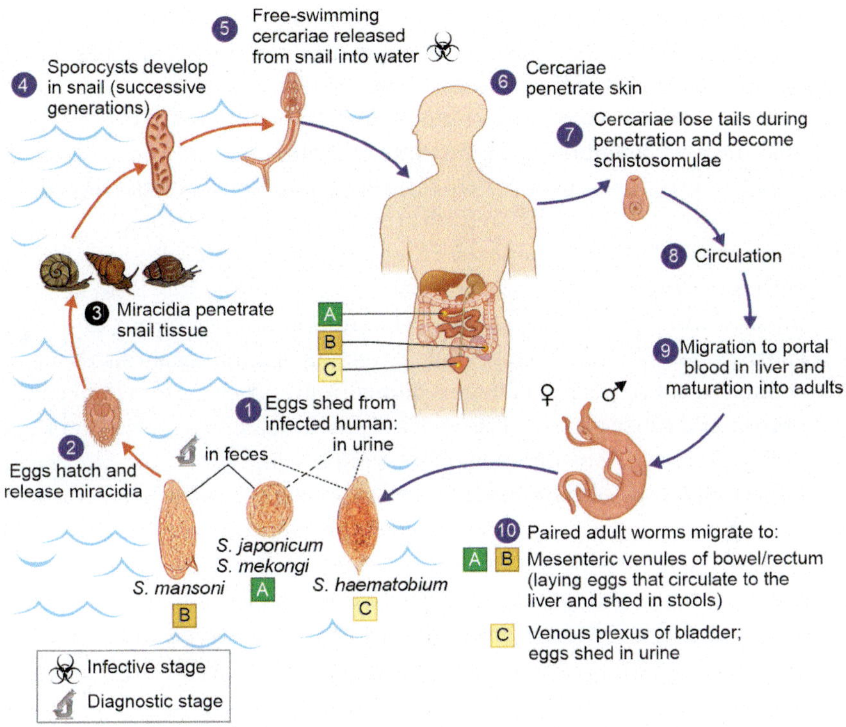

Fig. 1: Life cycle of *Schistosoma* species.
Source: CDC. Schistosomiasis. [online] Available from https://www.cdc.gov/dpdx/schistosomiasis/modules/Schistomes_LifeCycle_lg.jpg [Last accessed November, 2024].

fresh water. *Cercariae* acts as an infective form to human, the definitive host. **Figure 1** shows the life cycle of *Schistosoma*.

CLINICAL MANIFESTATIONS

Schistosomiasis occurs due to body's immune reaction to the eggs of the parasite. It may be asymptomatic in some individuals. Some patients present with small, pruritic, and maculopapular lesions which develops as a result of local cutaneous hypersensitivity reaction to entry of *Cercaria* in the body called "Swimmer's itch." A new clinical phase begins with the initiation of oviposition of *Schistosoma* eggs which include fever, chills, nausea, vomiting, urticaria, sweating, cough, abdominal pain, diarrhea, lymphadenopathy, and hepatosplenomegaly known as "Katayama fever" developing as a result of systemic hypersensitivity reaction to *Schistosoma* antigen, antigen like eggs that occurs several weeks after infection.[2,3] These symptoms resolve spontaneously in some days.

Chronic schistosomiasis have symptoms which correlate with the site in which eggs are trapped and the number of eggs in tissues and the immune response of host tissue. Intestinal schistosomiasis occurs with *S. mansoni* and *S. japonicum* as the eggs are released near the intestine resulting in symptoms like abdominal pain, intermittent diarrhea, and dysentery. Some may develop chronic colonic ulceration if the egg burden is too high leading to bleeding and anemia. Granulomatous inflammation may occur around eggs trapped in bowel wall which can cause intestinal polyps, intestinal dysplasia, bowel strictures or rarely obstruction, and appendicitis.

- *Hepatosplenic schistosomiasis:* In adolescents and children infected with *S. mansoni* and *japonicum*, nonfibrotic granulomas form around presinusoidal periportal spaces causing hepatomegaly but does not cause portal block and is reversible if treated. Splenomegaly also occurs. In adults, there occurs collagen deposition and granulomas become fibrotic and cause periportal fibrosis eventually leading to portal blockage and portal hypertension known as "Symmers pipestem fibrosis." Portal hypertension results in gastric and esophageal varices. Symptoms of hematemesis, jaundice, ascites, and hepatic failure develop in some.
- *Urinary schistosomiasis:* In *S. haematobium* infection, hematuria is seen due to excretion of eggs from perivesical plexus into urine. In early stages of chronic disease, granulomas form around eggs, inflammation occurs leading to ulceration and polyp formation. With time, bladder wall and ureters undergo fibrosis as a result of collagen deposition in granulomas and cause bladder neck obstruction. Dysuria, hydroureter, hydronephrosis, pyelonephritis, and renal failure may develop.[4]
- *Genital schistosomiasis:* Fallopian tubes involvement causes salpingitis and may cause infertility. Vulva, vagina, and cervix can get involved which causes ulceration and hypertrophy leading to dyspareunia.[5]
- *Pulmonary schistosomiasis:* Schistosoma eggs can embolize to pulmonary circulation due to portosystemic collaterals formed as a result of portal hypertension. These can lead to granulomatous pulmonary endarteritis leading to pulmonary hypertension and cor pulmonale. Symptoms of dyspnea, cough, and wheeze may occur and chest X-ray (CXR) shows fine military nodules.
- *Neuro-schistosomiasis:* Patients can get single or multiple space-occupying lesion or multifocal encephalopathy leading to sensory as well as motor deficiencies. Spinal cord may get involved leading to transverse myelitis like syndrome.

DIAGNOSIS AND TREATMENT

Microscopy

Schistosoma eggs are visualized in feces or urine in direct wet mount or after using concentration methods like formalin ethyl acetate. **Figure 2** shows the eggs of *Schistosoma mansoni*.

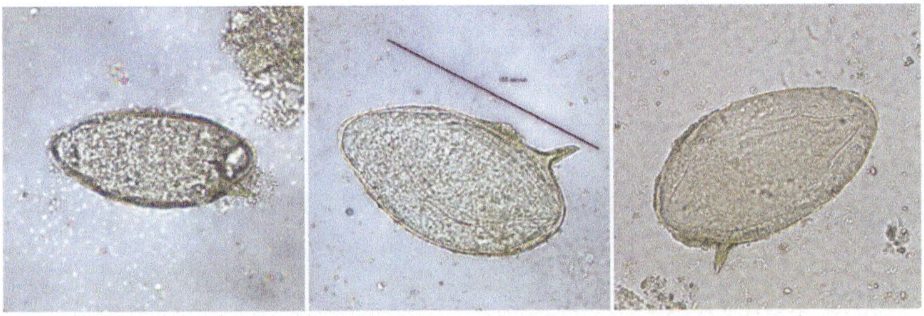

Fig. 2: Eggs of *Schistosoma mansoni* in an unstained wet mount.
Source: CDC. Schistosomiasis. [online] Available from https://www.cdc.gov/dpdx/schistosomiasis/ [Last accessed November, 2024].
Courtesy: Wisconsin State Laboratory of Hygiene, Missouri State Public Health Laboratory.

Molecular testing with polymerase chain reaction (PCR) to be undertaken if there is high suspicion of infection and microscopy exam is negative. Sample include serum, feces, urine, and cerebrospinal fluid (CSF).

Serologic tests: Antibody detection with the help of purified adult worm antigen can be done.

Blood test: Eosinophilia—30–60%, anemia, thrombocytopenia.

Therapy to be deferred until after pregnancy. *Praziquantel* 60 mg/kg PO in three divided doses for 1 day for *S. japonicum* and 40 mg/kg PO in two divided doses for one day in all other species of *Schistosoma*.

REFERENCES

1. Mahmoud AA. Current concepts: Schistosomiasis. N Engl J Med. 1977; 297(24):1329-31.
2. Warren KS. The pathology, pathobiology and pathogenesis of schistosomiasis. Nature. 1978;273(5664):609-12.
3. Young SW, Higashi G, Kamel R, el-Abdin AZ, Mikhail IA. Interaction of salmonellae and schistosomes in host parasite relations. Trans R Soc Trop Med Hyg. 1973;67(6):979.
4. Cowper SG. A Synopsis of African Bilharziasis. London: HK Lewis; 1971.
5. Gelfand M, Ross MD, Blair DM, Weber MC. Distribution and extent of schistosomiasis in female pelvic organs with special reference to the genital tract, as determined at autopsy. Am J Trop Med Hyg. 1971;20:846-9.

CHAPTER 11

Infection with Cestodes

INTRODUCTION

Tapeworms are widespread throughout the globe and resides in gastrointestinal tract of man. Disease causing tapeworms are *Taenia saginata, Taenia* solium, *Diphyllobothrium latum*, and *Hymenolepis nana*. Raw or uncooked beef or pork ingestion is the main cause of infection thus disease is common in areas like Europe and some parts of Asia where raw meat is eaten.

Adult worms are hermaphrodites, have a head or scolex containing hooks or suckers through which they attach to intestinal cells, neck, and a segmented body with each segment called proglottid and consisting of their own reproductive system.

Each species has their own morphologic characteristic which help in their identification. In *T. saginata,* scolex contain four lateral suckers without any hook so called unarmed, while *T. soilum* have a scolex which consist of a well-developed Rostellum with four suckers and two row of hooks. *D. latum* is the largest human tapeworm consisting of two bilateral sucking grooves on the scolex. **Figure 1** shows the life cycle of *Taenia* species.

Intermediate hosts consume eggs and larvae aka cysticerci develop into them which are also infective to another host if consumed. Intermediate host is cattle for *T. saginata* while pigs and humans in *T. soilum*. Crustacean and fish are the two intermediate host for *D. latum*. Sheep or cattle acts as an intermediate host for *E. granulosus* whereas dog is the definitive host and man as an accidental host.

CLINICAL MANIFESTATIONS

T. saginata: Infection is mostly asymptomatic while some presents with nausea, headache, anxiety, urticarial, anorexia, or epigastric pain. Passage of proglottids in feces may occur. Rarely, proglottids migrate to appendix or common bile duct or pancreatic duct and may cause obstruction.

T solium: T. soilum affects in the same way as *T. saginata*. Additionally, *T. solium* larvae causes cysticercosis in human tissues such as brain, muscle, or other tissue. Neurocysticercosis causes headache, papilledema, seizures, visual impairment, or hemiparesis. Cysticercosis occurs after ingestion of contaminated food containing *T. solium* eggs of the body. CNS involvement is common, and causes convulsions occasionally.

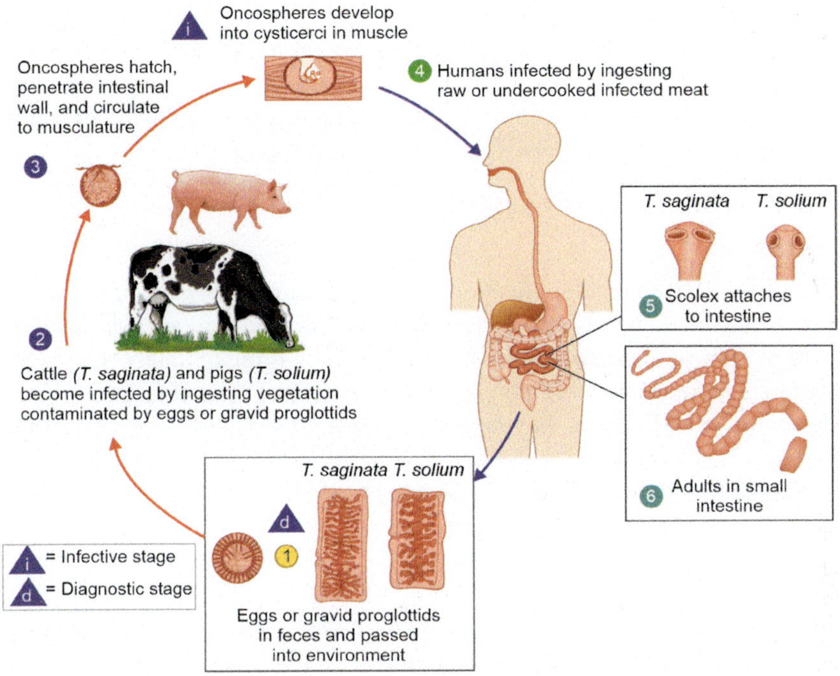

Fig. 1: Life cycle of *Taenia* species.
Source: CDC. Taeniasis. [online] Available from https://www.cdc.gov/dpdx/taeniasis/ https://www.cdc.gov/parasites/taeniasis/biology.html [Last accessed November, 2024].

D. latum: Most patients are asymptomatic or have mild abdominal discomfort. *D. latum* disintegrates vitamin B_{12} and intrinsic factor complex leading to reduced absorption of vitamin B_{12} and folic acid. Thus leading to megaloblastic anemia and symptoms of anemia such as fatigue, pallor, angular glossitis, stomatitis, papillary loss in tongue, irritability, and dizziness may occur. Numbness, paresthesia, loss of vibration sense, weakness, and unstable gait are all neurological manifestations due to vitamin B_{12} deficiency.

H. nana: Disease mostly occurs in children, is usually asymptomatic but during heavy infection with >1,000 worms patient show symptoms such as abdominal cramps, diarrhea, anorexia, irritability, dizziness, anemia, weight loss, fatigue, jaundice, or seizures.

E. granulosus: Disease is usually asymptomatic with long incubation period. Symptoms depend on the site where cyst develops. Usually one single cyst develops in most patients. Liver is most frequently involved with right lobe involvement more common than the left. Cyst may become very large, may rupture or remain dormant. Rupture of the cyst into peritoneum causes acute anaphylactic shock leading to multiple organ dysfunction syndrome (MODS) while rupture into biliary tree causes biliary colic, obstructive jaundice, or cholangitis or pancreatitis. Hydatid cyst can also rupture through the diaphragm into pleural space causing pleural effusion or pulmonary hydatidosis. Pulmonary involvement causes cough, chest pain, hemoptysis, or secondary bacterial infection may occur.

DIAGNOSIS AND TREATMENT

Microscopy

Diagnosis is based on identification and visualization of eggs or proglottid in feces with the help of special stain like India ink. For cysticercosis, X-ray of skull or computed tomography (CT) scan can be done to detect the lesion. MRI may be required to demonstrate live cysticercal cysts **(Fig. 2)**. **Figure 3** shows unstained eggs of *Taenia* spp. **Figure 4** shows adult worm of *Taenia saginata*.

Coproantigen or molecular assay are more sensitive but not routinely used. Serologic tests for research settings.

Treatment

Praziquantal is the mainstay of treatment in tapeworm diseases dose being 5–10 mg/kg PO single dose. Praziquantal and niclosamide are pregnancy category B drugs. Alternative drug which can be used are niclosamide or albendazole. Niclosamide at a dose of 2 g PO single dose. Albendazole at a dose 400 mg OD for 3 days can also be used. For neurocysticercosis, focus is on symptomatic management such as seizure control and intracranial

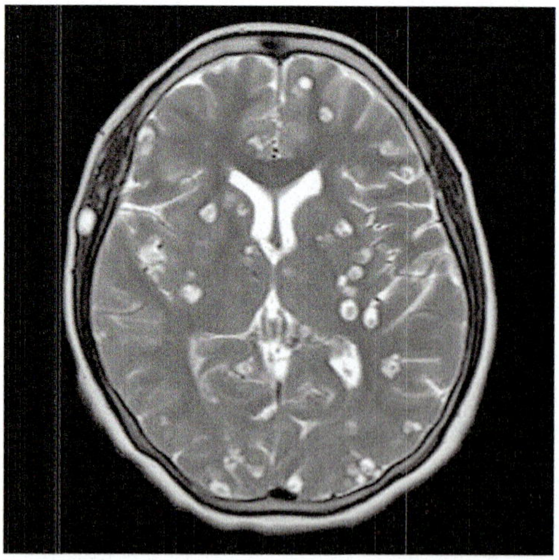

Fig. 2: Live cysticercal cysts on T2 weighted (T2W) magnetic resource imaging (MRI) of the brain. Note the scolex within the cysts seen as a "cyst with dot sign."
Source: Gaillard F, Weerakkody Y. (2021). Neurocysticercosis. [online] Available from https://radiopaedia.org/articles/1724 [Last accessed November, 2024].

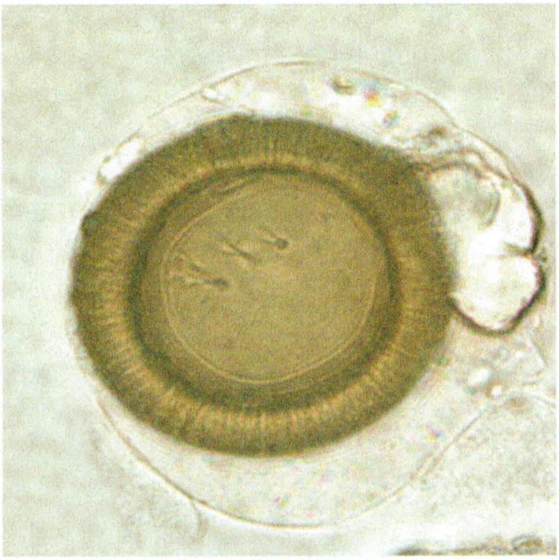

Fig. 3: Unstained *Taenia* spp. egg. Four hooks can easily be seen in this image.
Source: CDC website. Taenia egg. [online] Available from https://www.cdc.gov/dpdx/taeniasis/images/1/Taenia_egg1.jpg [Last accessed November, 2024].

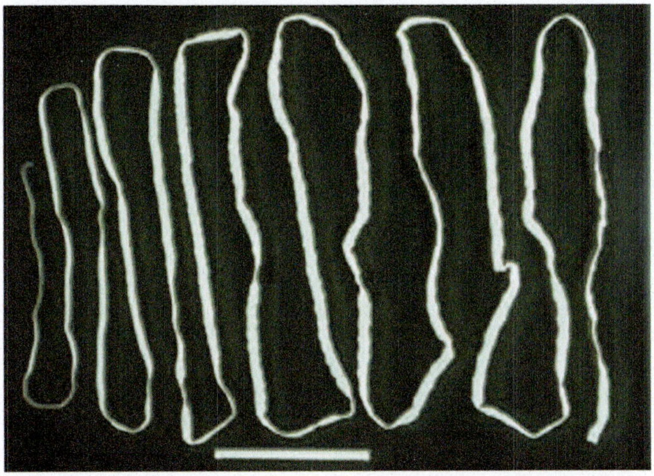

Fig. 4: *Taenia saginata* adult worm. The adult in this image is approximately 4 meters in length.
Source: CDC. Taenia saginata. [online] Available from https://www.cdc.gov/dpdx/taeniasis/images/5/Taenia_saginata_adult1.jpg [Last accessed November, 2024].

hypertension correction. Ventricular shunt and other neurosurgical procedures may be used. Corticosteroids like dexamethasone should be given if anthelminthic therapy instituted in these patients. Hydatid disease is also treated surgically with removal of cyst en-sac. High-dose mebendazole can be administered to kill larval forms **(Fig. 2)**.

Treatment of intestinal tapeworms, including *T. saginata, T. solium,* and *D. latum,* is praziquantel 10–20 mg/kg in a single dose. Treatment of *H. nana* also is a single dose of praziquantel 25 mg/kg. Alternative therapy is niclosamide 2 g chewed thoroughly, then 1 g/day (two tablets) for 6 days. Treatment of cysticercosis or hydatid disease is based on surgical removal of the intact cyst if it is inducing obstructive symptoms. Care should be exercised in preventing spillage of the cyst contents into the peritoneum. Several studies have suggested that high-dose mebendazole administration is effective in killing tapeworms in the larval stage. This treatment is useful for patients who cannot undergo surgery or as adjunctive therapy.

12 CHAPTER Multiple Choice Questions

1. **A 28-year-old pregnant woman in her first trimester presents to the clinic with a history of handling cat litter without gloves. She is concerned about her risk for toxoplasmosis, as she recently read that it can affect her baby. She reports mild flu-like symptoms and has no other significant medical history. What is the most appropriate next step for diagnosing toxoplasmosis in this pregnant woman?**
   a. Ultrasound to check for fetal anomalies
   b. Serological testing for toxoplasmosis immunoglobulin M (IgM) and immunoglobulin G (IgG) antibodies
   c. Amniocentesis to test for toxoplasmosis in the fetus
   d. Immediate treatment with pyrimethamine and sulfadiazine

Ans. b. Serological testing for toxoplasmosis immunoglobulin M (IgM) and immunoglobulin G (IgG) antibodies

2. **A 30-year-old pregnant woman at 12 weeks of gestation complains of persistent diarrhea, abdominal cramps, and bloating. She recently returned from a camping trip where she drank untreated water from a stream. A stool sample reveals the presence of *Giardia lamblia*. What is the most appropriate treatment for giardiasis during pregnancy?**
   a. Metronidazole
   b. Tinidazole
   c. Albendazole
   d. Paromomycin

Ans. d. Paromomycin

3. **A 28-year-old pregnant woman, at 30 weeks of gestation, presents with fever, chills, fatigue, and headache after returning from a trip to a malaria-endemic region in Southeast Asia. Laboratory results reveal a positive rapid diagnostic test (RDT) for *Plasmodium falciparum* and the following abnormalities:**

   ***Hemoglobin:* 8.0 g/dL**

   ***Platelet count:* 100,000/μL**

   ***Liver enzymes (AST/ALT):* mildly elevated**

   ***Peripheral blood smear: Plasmodium falciparum* trophozoites and schizonts seen**

   No signs of severe malaria (e.g., no cerebral malaria, hypoglycemia, or severe anemia)

What is the most appropriate first-line treatment for this patient, considering both the safety of the pregnancy and the severity of the malaria infection?

a. Artemisinin-based combination therapy (ACT)—artemether-lumefantrine
b. Quinine and clindamycin
c. Mefloquine
d. Chloroquine and primaquine

Ans. b. Quinine and clindamycin

4. **A pregnant woman at 16 weeks of gestation is diagnosed with *Schistosoma mansoni* infection after traveling to an endemic area. She is asymptomatic, but the diagnosis was made based on routine screening. What is the most appropriate approach for treating schistosomiasis in this pregnancy?**

a. Initiate treatment with praziquantel immediately after diagnosis.
b. Treatment will be delayed until after the second trimester.
c. Monitor the patient closely, and treat only if symptoms develop.
d. Treat with albendazole in the first trimester.

Ans. a. Initiate treatment with praziquantel immediately after diagnosis.

5. **A 22-year-old pregnant woman at 24 weeks of gestation with a history of *Schistosoma haematobium* infection presents for her routine antenatal visit. What additional management should be provided to this patient besides treatment for schistosomiasis?**

a. Iron supplementation for anemia prevention
b. High-dose corticosteroids to reduce inflammation
c. Bed rest to prevent pregnancy complications
d. No additional management is needed if the infection is treated

Ans. a. Iron supplementation for anemia prevention

6. **Which parasitic infection is associated with anemia and bloody diarrhea in pregnancy, commonly contracted by drinking contaminated water?**

a. Toxoplasmosis
b. Giardiasis
c. Hookworm
d. Schistosomiasis

Ans. b. Giardiasis

7. **The most common parasitic cause of microcephaly and hydrocephalus in pregnancy is:**

a. Toxoplasmosis
b. Malaria
c. Schistosomiasis
d. Trichomoniasis

Ans. a. Toxoplasmosis

8. A 28-year-old pregnant woman at 16 weeks of gestation presents with concern about toxoplasmosis after handling raw meat and cleaning her cat's litter box. Her serology shows IgG-positive and IgM-negative. What does this finding indicate?

a. Recent infection with toxoplasmosis
b. Past infection with toxoplasmosis
c. Active infection with toxoplasmosis
d. No risk of toxoplasmosis infection

Ans. b. Past infection with toxoplasmosis

9. Which of the following is the most important prevention strategy for toxoplasmosis in pregnancy?

a. Avoiding consumption of undercooked meat
b. Using pyrimethamine during pregnancy
c. Avoiding contact with soil
d. Avoiding contact with infected animals only

Ans. a. Avoiding consumption of undercooked meat

10. Which of the following is the treatment of choice for acute toxoplasmosis in pregnancy, particularly if the infection is diagnosed in the second or third trimester?

a. Pyrimethamine and sulfadiazine
b. Albendazole
c. Mebendazole
d. Praziquantel

Ans. a. Pyrimethamine and sulfadiazine

11. A pregnant woman tests positive for *Toxoplasma* IgM and IgG antibodies. What is the next best step in management?

a. Start treatment with pyrimethamine and sulfadiazine
b. Perform amniocentesis for fetal infection
c. Repeat serology in 4 weeks
d. Begin iron supplementation to prevent anemia

Ans. b. Perform amniocentesis for fetal infection

12. A 29-year-old pregnant woman at 22 weeks of gestation is diagnosed with *Plasmodium falciparum* malaria. Which of the following is the most likely complication if left untreated?

a. Neonatal jaundice
b. Fetal anemia
c. Congenital malformations
d. Fetal death

Ans. b. Fetal anemia

13. A 35-year-old pregnant woman with a history of hookworm infection presents with fatigue, pallor, and poor appetite. What is the most likely complication for the fetus?

a. Intrauterine growth restriction (IUGR)
b. Preterm labor

c. Fetal anemia
d. Fetal hydrops

Ans. a. Intrauterine growth restriction (IUGR)

14. A pregnant woman at 22 weeks of gestation presents with complaints of watery diarrhea, fatigue, and bloating after traveling to an area with poor sanitation. She is diagnosed with giardiasis. What is the most likely route of transmission?

a. Fecal-oral transmission through contaminated food or water
b. Inhalation of contaminated dust particles
c. Contact with infected pets
d. Sexual transmission

Ans. a. Fecal-oral transmission through contaminated food or water

15. Which of the following is the best management for a pregnant woman with a hookworm infection during the first trimester?

a. Immediate albendazole treatment
b. Iron supplementation and delay deworming until the second trimester
c. Mebendazole for the first 12 weeks
d. Praziquantel for effective treatment

Ans. b. Iron supplementation and delay deworming until the second trimester

Index

Page numbers followed by *f* refer to figure, and *t* refer to table.

F

G

H

I

K

L

M

N

O

P

R

S